I Got Cancer,
But Cancer Didn't Get Me

To:
Jim Ritchay   Stay Strong!
A fellow warrior in the
fight against cancer.
Health & Happiness Always!
Remember, Together We
Can STINGCANCER!

I Got Cancer, But Cancer Didn't Get Me

The Story of My Cancer Journey and the Birth of STINGCANCER

Cover photos by Mike Roemer, Mike Roemer Photography Inc.

ISBN-13: 978-0-9960488-1-1

ISBN-10: 0996048812

Published by M&B Global Solutions Inc.
United States of America (USA)

I Got Cancer, But Cancer Didn't Get Me

*The Story of My Cancer Journey
and the Birth of STINGCANCER*

By Nick Nesvacil

Accolades

"Nick's story will provide inspiration and hope for anyone going through their own cancer journey."

Jerry Parins, author of "Bodyguard to the Packers: Beat Cops, Brett Favre and Beating Cancer"

"While there are many stories of success in battling cancer, Nick's story is one of relentless courage coupled with a determination to live that is far greater than anyone I have ever met. He is the epitome of "Never, ever, give up!" and his journey is one for the research books. Most of all, it's what Nick does with this rejuvenated life that is amazing."

David Yates, author of "Cancer Sucks - A True Story"

Dedication

This book is gratefully dedicated to my dad, without whom I could not have survived; and to my family today, who remind me every day the reason I survived.

Acknowledgements

I would like to thank God for allowing me extra time on this amazing earth to meet unbelievable people and follow all my dreams.

I want to thank my Dad, who was always my rock and will always be a huge reason why I am a survivor.

I want to thank Dr. Tadanori Tomita for performing the surgery that saved my life when no one else could.

I want to thank Jerry Parins and the Green Bay Packers for acknowledging and supporting the accomplishments of STINGCANCER, and giving me the confidence to keep building it into what it is today.

I want to thank Dr. Chris Wagner for allowing me to start STINGCANCER at Preble High School when neither of us knew if a cancer awareness group would work in a school setting.

I want to thank all the amazing STINCANCER advisors and at-large members over the last eleven years. You are the reason why STINGCANCER has turned into a powerful group in more than twenty schools so far.

I would like to thank Mike Dauplaise and Amy Mrotek for helping me write a book that we hope will inspire many.

I would like to thank Mike Daniels and Nicolet Bank for supporting STINGCANCER in so many ways.

I would like to thank all my amazing friends and family members who are the reason I am here today.

I would like to thank all the amazing people who have battled cancer in one way or another. You make up such an amazing network of people.

I would like to thank everyone who has made up the Preble building over the last eleven years. Without your amazing support, STINGCANCER would not be what it is today.

Most of all, I would like to say thank you to my five miracles: my wife, Maureen; and children Grace, Claire, Evelyn and Nicholas. You are the best family ever and make me a better person every day.

Contents

Preface 11

Chapter 1 – Two "C-Words" I Could Not Say 17

Chapter 2 – Growing Up 27

Chapter 3 – Football and the Green Bay Packers 41

Chapter 4 – My Dad 57

Chapter 5 – The Value of Friends 63

Chapter 6 – The Effects of Brain Cancer 77

Chapter 7 – Surviving Cancer 87

Chapter 8 – My Life After Cancer 97

Chapter 9 – Making a Difference 101

Chapter 10 – Starting Your Own STINGCANCER Group 121

STINGCANCER Testimonials 129

About the Author 139

Preface

I remember as a child thinking about the legend of the boogeyman. I always wondered if there truly was a boogeyman who jumped out of the closet and scared the life out of you. I'll never forget that cold, dark, lonely Saturday night when I felt like a prisoner in a Chicago hospital. All my friends and family had retired for the night. It was just me, the clock, and the harsh reality that I had brain cancer.

The boogeyman had jumped out of the closet that night in the form of cancer, and I was more scared than I could ever remember. Those three words – "You have cancer" – are some of the most powerful and frightening words anyone can ever hear. Just weeks earlier, I would have been having a beer with my football buddies or out to eat with my girlfriend on just such a night. Not anymore. Cancer had entered my life and it would never be the same.

Earlier in the day, I had recollections of people whispering, taking part in private conversations. I'm sure that was to protect me from the truth, but all it did was scare me more. As I lay there, a million thoughts went through my mind. More surgery? Chemotherapy? Radiation? Physical therapy? Occupational therapy? Speech therapy? What was happening? Cancer was happening.

And at that time in that lonely bed, watching that lonely clock, I could not do a damn thing about it. One thing I learned early on with my cancer is you can sit and feel sorry for yourself as long as you want, but you won't see any positive results from doing that. No matter how terrible I felt because of my appearance – the lazy eye, the scarred, bald head, the complete loss of balance when walking, being sixty pounds lighter – I learned quickly that if I did not change my feelings about myself, I would be unable to change my outward actions toward others.

If I was going to survive cancer, I needed to have all my friends and family in my corner. Feeling sorry for myself was not an option. It's like when you're playing cards: You must accept the cards dealt to you; but ultimately, you choose how to play the hand.

Every thought a survivor has shapes their journey. I have a saying on my classroom door where I teach: "Our thoughts become our words. Our words become our actions. Our actions become our habits. Our habits become our character. Our character becomes our destiny. And our destiny ultimately becomes our legacy." It is important for me to always remember the importance of leaving a positive legacy.

Attitude is so important in the battle with cancer. It is the difference between one person with cancer thriving and another giving up. Cancer happened to me. *I got cancer, but cancer didn't get me!* It comes down to while we may not *have* the best of everything, we need to do what we can to *make* the best of everything. Many medical professionals have observed a positive correlation between people's attitudes and their ability to recover from illness.

In this book, I will use my story to illustrate the importance that attitude, support systems and goals have in the fight against cancer. I will also provide a template you can follow to support cancer patients and their families in your community.

Perhaps you are in the midst of the fight of your life. It's natural to struggle with fear and the fact there is so little within your control regarding your physical health. I know. I've been there. However, you can choose to control virtually everything associated with your mental health, and believe it or not, that definitely carries over to your physical recovery.

My hope is my story and the tools I share will help you come through the other side with a new lease on life. Not necessarily the same life, but perhaps an even better one than you have ever imagined. I know that was the case with me.

Author Chuck Swindoll said, "I am convinced that life is 10 percent what happens to me and 90 percent how I react to it. Our attitude is ultimately our emotional approach to life, and if we do not have a positive one, we sure are not helping ourselves."

My thought at that time was beating cancer was not impossible. While it was never easy, I believe my attitude was a difference-maker in my battle against cancer. I call it a difference-maker because it has helped me open doors and overcome obstacles since the day I was diagnosed.

My attitude toward cancer has allowed me to become a teacher, a football coach and the founder and advisor of STINGCANCER. This group is my proudest achievement. STINGCANCER started out as a small social group at Green Bay (Wisconsin) Preble High School to discuss cancer. It has evolved into a powerful cancer awareness group powered by students in more than twenty schools in Northeast Wisconsin as of this writing.

Having a great attitude does not mean cancer is fun or simple. It is easy to allow a huge change in your life, such as cancer, to affect you negatively. You can allow change to get the best of you or you can harness change and let it play a role in making the best of you. Our perspective on something like cancer, rather than the cancer itself, can help determine our outcome. It is important to remember the size of the person is more important than the size of the problem. Big people overcome big obstacles.

In fact, that is why cancer survivors are some of the strongest, most dynamic people I have ever met. It is probably because many of these people would not be so driven to succeed without having gone through the challenges cancer brought to their life. I know for a fact the challenges cancer presented to me are the very things that drove me to start STINGCANCER and make a difference in the world. They say that adversity paves the way for success, and my struggle with cancer is the chip on my shoulder.

The battle against cancer is no doubt intimidating. Taking action against cancer definitely has its risks and costs. They are far less, however, than the risks and costs of not taking action. Fear robs a lot of us of our potential to fight against cancer. Fear of recurrence still is a huge dread of mine. The key is to focus on our faith and continually feed it. I believe cancer patients gain strength, courage and confidence through every experience in which we stop to look fear in the face.

People who gain momentum in refusing to quit and finding success against their cancer develop an attitude of tenacity. I know tenacity raged inside of me as I felt compelled to prove to everyone that I made it, that I beat cancer. Every person who has ever achieved anything really significant has had to overcome the odds. My achievements include my wonderful family, my great job as a teacher, a master's degree and being the founder of

STINGCANCER. What are your amazing achievements in life? We all have them.

Whether you are a cancer survivor, have a loved one battling cancer, or you have been hit by a different kind of roadblock in the crazy life we all live, this book will open your mind to realize that you, too, are a strong survivor. With the right attitude and a little tenacity, you can get through anything.

Chapter 1

Two "C-Words" I Could Not Say

Almost overnight, the words cancer and chemotherapy became constants in the vocabulary used by people in my inner circle. I refused to take part in this self-defeating nonsense. I literally could not say the words cancer or chemotherapy. The idea of me having cancer and going through chemotherapy was ludicrous.

I decided that I would tell my friends and the people around me I was sick and undergoing treatment. While the only person I was fooling was me, it made me feel better about my situation in the beginning. Those in my inner circle knew what was happening, but when I would run into someone I had not seen in a while, it made me feel better to leave out chemo and cancer and any other specifics I did not want to share.

Looking back, I must have looked like a fool. However, it was all simply impossible for me to accept. Nobody needed to know that a former college football player and a dean's list student was now going through cancer and receiving some of the harshest chemotherapy and radiation known to man. Those words simply would not come out of my mouth. I felt already defeated by saying them. My family knew, my few very close friends knew. But as far as I was concerned, nobody else needed to know. I was ignorant enough to think this cancer thing was going to be a short-term roadblock and, just maybe, I could pull a fast one on people not in my inner circle.

When I eventually got to the point where I wanted to educate myself more on those words, I only became more frightened. I looked up cancer in the Merriam-Webster Dictionary, and it read: "Cancer: a malignant tumor of potentially limited growth that expands locally by invasion and systematically by metastasis or an abnormal bodily state marked by tumors."

Then I proceeded to look up chemotherapy, and it read: "Chemotherapy: refers to drugs that are used to kill microorganisms or the use of chemical agents in the treatment or control of a disease or mental illness."

These two descriptions were not exactly the ringing endorsements I was looking for. I then found out that while surgery and radiation therapy destroy or damage cancer cells in a specific area, chemotherapy works throughout the whole body. So it would not only try to kill the malignant tumor in my brain, but it would also do its best to try to kill me over the next sixteen weeks.

After reading the American Cancer Society's description of how chemotherapy works, my only question was, "What would the chemo kill first? The cancer or me?"

My doctors told me because I was young and otherwise healthy, they were going to be especially aggressive with my chemo treatments. This is when I started to realize that I was in for a long, bumpy ride. My oncologist told me my treatment plan would be sixteen weeks long. I would have one full week of chemo and then need three weeks to recover. I would have four rounds of this one-week-on-and-three-weeks-off cycle.

I thought I was over the most difficult obstacle after seven weeks in the hospital and four surgical procedures. I was wrong. My life suddenly consisted of a reclining chair, a stale can of Sprite® and a long intravenous (IV) drip that became my worst enemy.

The goal of chemotherapy is to destroy cancer cells. Traditional chemotherapies work by killing cells that divide rapidly. As they wipe out fast-growing cancer cells, though, they can also damage fast-growing healthy cells. Damage to blood cells, for example, leads to side effects such as anemia, fatigue and infections.

Chemotherapy can also damage the cells that line the mucous membranes found throughout the body, including those inside the mouth, throat and stomach. This leads to mouth sores, diarrhea, or other problems with the digestive system. Damaging cells at hair roots, or hair follicles, leads to hair loss.

While I experienced much of this physical damage, what was going on emotionally was even worse. A typical day for chemo treatment was my dad waking me up at around 7 a.m.. If you think it is hard getting up for work or school, this is a whole different animal.

My dad was awesome. He would gently coax me out of bed as I continued to resist. When I finally got up, I had breakfast with a chaser of anti-nausea medication that had be taken at least an hour before the chemo started. I was in no hurry. It's not like I was going to a concert or a great night out. It's not like they could start without me.

On the way to the hospital, my mind would deal with this terrifying fact: the only way my doctor can think of to totally cure me is to inject poison into my system – in a controlled, hygienic way, of course. The poison will kill not only my cancer cells, but also a lot of other things: my hair cells, those lining my mouth, and the good bacteria in my gut.

Chemotherapy is boring; not a bang, but a whimper. You sit in your recliner all day, tethered to a pole from which hang several bags of fluids containing your chemo drugs. Movement is restricted to bathroom breaks, which are a comic dance of you and the pole on wheels, and all the cords connecting your IV to them. You will take the chemo home with you, of course, carrying it in your gut and your veins. Over the next few days, your body will slowly eliminate it. Your pee will smell funny. You will take the steroids home as well. They may induce sleeplessness and manic energy.

Throughout my journey with chemo, I felt emotions such as shock. I wanted to know what was happening. How did I end up here? I went through denial. This could not be happening to me. I was invincible. I experienced bitterness. Why were all my friends out enjoying themselves and I was fighting for my life? In many ways, I felt guilty. What did I do to make this happen? How did I cause my cancer and put myself in this situation? Was I being punished for something?

My mom died when I was twelve. I had just experienced a brutal knee injury from football a few months earlier. I was still recovering from multiple brain surgeries, a stroke and a life-threatening infection. Did I really deserve to now face this poison that was going to kill whatever was left of me?

Chemo sessions ran for a week of treatment, where I would sit in a recliner from 8 a.m. until noon, Monday through Friday, and watch this horrible liquid drip into my body. I remember the calm before the storm being the worst; the time before I landed in that recliner. All the things that happened from the time my dad dragged me out of bed to when I landed in that chair are still very vivid.

I remember the long, barren brick hallway I had to walk down to the oncology unit. It smelled like an old, deserted building. The hallway itself looked and felt like it had been deserted for years. The first things that came to mind were must and mold. Couldn't someone have provided some air fresheners or something? Nothing about this walk was inviting in any way. It was so cold and isolating that it seemed to almost take my breath away.

Looking back, it seemed like a prison. Seeing how my immune system and spirits were already at an all-time low, couldn't the hospital have made this path to treatment a bit more welcoming? I mean, I had just dodged death once, and now I was tempting fate by being on this journey to chemotherapy, which it seemed was trying to kill me again.

The best analogy I can think of is this: remember when you were a little kid, preparing to jump in really cold water? I remember after a few seconds in the water, everything was okay. The water felt warm and all was good. As I felt the same trepidation entering my chemo sessions, the result was much different. That frigid chill that went away after jumping in the cold water wasn't the same with chemotherapy. That frigid chill of this therapy lasted for those four grueling hours while I sat in that recliner. As I sat there, many different people of all ages, shapes, sexes, etc., came through.

I remember the first day. Everyone seemed to be at least three times my age. They seemed to have nothing in common with me. Oh yeah, except for the fact they had cancer and were fighting for their lives just like I was. The whole scene in the beginning made me bitter. I was mad that I had cancer and now I was really mad that I was going through chemotherapy with people way older than me. What did I do to deserve this? It was the most awkward, unwelcoming experience I had ever felt.

Once I got home, that cold feeling turned to overwhelming exhaustion. I went to sleep for a long time. This was partly because of how much the chemo had depleted my system and partly because when I was sleeping, I was not thinking about having cancer.

Eventually, after waking up, I felt like I had the worst flu epidemic known to man. Only when one gets the flu, it is typically for 24 to 48 hours. This flu-like feeling lasted about twenty weeks as the chemo invaded my body. As each chemo session added to the one before, my body and mind felt much worse.

I remember appreciating the smiles and greetings from the oncology staff each morning. But in the back of my mind, I knew they were just trying to lessen the harsh, hellish reality of what cancer and chemotherapy can do to a person.

This harsh reality included night pains in my stomach, side and back that kept me up many nights and caused me to be increasingly tired. I also experienced a lot of pain and uneasiness urinating due to all the chemicals that were filling my body. Occasionally, this was accompanied by urges to throw up just because I ate the wrong thing at the wrong time. I also had periods of diarrhea and lack of hunger that decreased my already-low weight.

The night pains you experience are painful. As you roll around in bed, you realize how this poison has affected every part of your physical being. These not only remained constant through my chemo sessions, but they lasted for years after my treatment was completed. My oncologist told me they were a normal side effect of chemotherapy.

Normal is a funny word. Nothing seems the least bit normal when your world is surrounded by the words cancer and chemotherapy.

My appetite sure was not normal. I had already lost about thirty pounds during my surgeries and extended hospital stay. The chemo had wiped out my appetite. This was a major concern for my survival. After the first two rounds of chemo, I had no initiative to eat or even smell food. Everything made me feel nauseous. I was losing more weight by the day. After multiple surgeries, multiple chemo treatments and a future date with sixteen weeks of radiation, I had now lost nearly sixty pounds.

My football playing weight was 215 pounds. Now I was down to about 155 and my immune system was shattered. The doctors decided from that point on, my chemo sessions would have to be on an inpatient basis and heavily monitored. I was a fragment of my former self.

At one point during my chemo treatment, I remember falling asleep on a Tuesday morning and not waking up until Friday afternoon. Nobody ever said I was in a coma, but that sure was what it felt like.

At this point, my attitude was at an all-time low. Aside from losing my eye brows and all body hair, having a lazy eye due to my stroke, numerous scars on my head, the weight loss and night pains that felt like someone was jabbing a sharp sword into my stomach and back, the bottom line was chemo sucked. It may have been killing the cancer cells in my brain, but at the same time I felt like it was going to kill me.

My attitude was exhausted. After all the surgeries, all the poking and prodding over the last six weeks, what I needed was a break. But aggressive cancer does not allow a break. Removing the tumor in my head was not enough. Now we had to kill any potential cancer cells that may be lingering near the spot of where the tumor was. This sucked. I was beat down. I had already been through hell and back, and now this treatment was like pouring salt on the wound. As my body began falling apart, so too was my attitude.

Why do we as a culture expect positivity from those on the other side of cancer treatment? Why do we demand an upbeat attitude from people who have seen the extremes of hardship or perpetuate this idea that there is a "right" way to suffer from a disease? There is no "right" way.

Because food was not my friend and my immune system and weight were so low, I was given a steroid to help me regain my appetite. This not only made me begin to consume about five full meals a day, but also made me look like a chipmunk on a steroid rage. Needless to say, I regained the weight I needed, but not in a particularly healthy way.

Steroids are the unsung heroes of cancer care. While chemo and radiation get all the accolades for killing cancer, steroids work quietly behind the scenes, preventing and minimizing complications and even making other therapies work better. I understand their importance in the battle against cancer, but I did not like the way they made me look or feel. I guess in the long run, I had to remember they helped me put on weight, rebuild my immune system and maybe they even kept me alive.

My dad helped me try anything to make this experience better. We tried more natural foods, visits to nutrition centers and even a few herbal remedies. They all helped somewhat, but eventually chemotherapy and its effects overcame all these things.

What ultimately got me through these sessions of poison intake were my close friends. My dad was my best friend. His steadying influence and constant support was what I leaned on the most. He was truly my rock. My siblings followed his lead and were always there for me.

My best friend, Darren, was always there for me. Many other friends would come and go. While they meant well, they usually stuck around, wished me their best and then left when things got awkward. Darren was different. It was like he had an innate sense of what I was thinking and even going through to a certain extent. He would come visit and just talk to me when I wanted to, and he sat quietly by my bed when I didn't want to talk. Many times he stayed by my side for hours when he had a lot of other things he could have been doing. To me, this was friendship at its best.

Even with endless support from family, friends and countless others, at the end of the day, the cancer chemo experience is one that takes tenacity from within and a strong ability to persevere. There had never been two more scary words in my life than cancer and chemotherapy.

During my chemo treatments, I began to realize the lives of everyone around me were going on as usual, regardless of what was happening with me. I was discovering that my previous life was gone. Ultimately, I had two choices: I could give up or rise up.

Even as chemotherapy came to an end, I began to realize my road to recovery was still only in the early stages. I was still facing eighteen weeks of radiation, half on the area where my tumor was in my head, and half down my brain stem for preventative reasons.

I also began six months of occupational, speech and physical therapy. Along with this, I was about to embark on a two-year relationship with a neuropsychologist to help me with memory, focus and concentration.

Less than a year before this journey, I was beginning to write my legacy as a dean's list student and college football player. What was it going to be now? A guy who got cancer and tried hard to beat it, but…

Chapter 2

Growing Up

I guess one could say I was a survivor even before I was born. My mom was four months pregnant in 1975. About a week after she announced this pregnancy to her older children, who were 17, 16, and 11, she had a miscarriage.

The crazy thing was even after the doctor gave my mom the pills needed to clean out her uterus, my mom had a funny feeling something was going on in her body. She went back for her six-week check-up after the miscarriage, convinced she was still pregnant. When she told her doctor her thoughts, he told her she was crazy and needed to get some rest. He insisted he had seen the fetal material during the miscarriage. Being pregnant was impossible.

However, my mom pointed to some freckle-like bumps on her neck that only appeared during her pregnancies. They were still there. It had been six weeks since her miscarriage. She convinced the doctor to feel her abdomen. That is when things got scary. He told my mom he was sure she had a tumor.

After many days of concern, my mom's doctor did an x-ray. They found no tumor. However, they did find me. Mom was right; there was something still in her belly: me!

My mom went on to have me six weeks early, and many people did not even know she was having a baby. I was around five pounds at birth, which was large compared to many of the premature babies in the NICU. My twin had died earlier, and somehow I remained and survived the medical procedure that took place after the miscarriage.

Today, I still have a bump on the back of my head caused by the cleaning-out, post-miscarriage process. Ironically, our doctor referred to me as a "tumor" when I was a child. Maybe that was a bad omen.

I remember seeing a story in a newspaper cutout my mom had from the *Guinness Book of World Records*. It was in reference to the time between a miscarriage and a healthy delivery of another baby. The woman who had the record was only about four days different than my mom. Absolutely crazy.

I was born to Nicholas J. Nesvacil and Maureen A. Nesvacil on October 11, 1975. I was not initially part of the Nesvacil family's plan. My oldest brother Jay was 17; my oldest sister Nancy was 16; and my youngest sister Nora was 11. All of the sudden, my mom was pregnant at age 42. She also battled Crohn's disease until the day she died.

My mom described me as a pleasant surprise and my dad, who was 46 at the time, jokingly dubbed me an accident. My mom was a hard-working first aide nurse at Fort Howard Paper Company in Green Bay, the largest paper mill in town. My dad also worked crazy hours as a truck driver for Green Bay Dressed Beef.

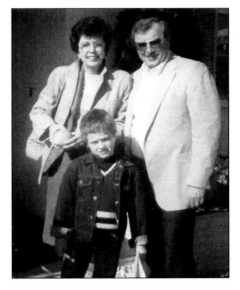

As a child, I did not have a normal relationship with my parents like most of my peers did with theirs. My mom and dad were often mistaken for my grandparents when we were in public. My dad and I did not do typical father-son activities; partially because he was constantly on the road working, but also because he was in his mid-fifties and not in the greatest physical shape when I needed him for those father-son type activities. Often I remember my older brother, Jay, stepping in for father-son Little League or Boy Scout events.

The best way to describe my mom was ultra-, sometimes even over-protective. Even though she was an educated nurse, she was extremely germophobic. I remember when a family member came home from a hospital visit or a doctor's appointment, they were immediately told to strip down and take a shower.

She had a fear that someone in our family was going to catch some terrible disease. Is it not ironic she died at age 54 of complications from Crohn's disease? I can't even imagine the conspiracy theories that she would have had regarding my brain cancer and how I contracted it.

Growing up was difficult in that my dad was always on the road, my siblings were young adults and moved out and my mom seemed to always be tired and/or sick. I really thought it sucked when I was young that I was the kid with the old mom and dad. When my mom died, that bitterness turned into more of a fear. I was only 13 years old. The anxiety of potentially being the only kid at school without living parents constantly ate at me.

I really believe my mom was left on earth just long enough to make sure I was on the straight and narrow path. She did so in a manner I often thought was harsh and hardcore, but looking back, I realize that it was all part of what has shaped me into the person I am today. I know my mom loved me more than anything, but when I was young it was hard to see it that way. When she would not let me do things, I never considered the fact that she was very ill. I often looked at it like she was only restricting me to make me mad.

Now that I am a parent of four, I can sympathize with my mom so much more. My mom refused to let me get away with anything. If all my friends could stay outside until 10 p.m. in the summer, she did not care. My curfew was still 9 p.m. If all my friends had bedtimes of 9 p.m. on school nights, mine was still 8 p.m. She never wavered in her rules, no matter how much I whined or complained.

It was almost like she knew she was not going to be around for all of my younger years and wanted to make sure she instilled proper morals and values in the short time she and I were on this earth together. She always set the standards for our family and stood by them at all costs.

One of the hardest things for me is I do not remember as much about my mom as I'd like to. With her being gone now more than twenty-five years and me having a very sketchy memory, it is hard to remember as much as I'd like to about her.

I do remember that she always worried about me in public. She feared that I would get lost or taken by somebody. My dad would tell her, "Don't worry, Maureen. If anyone takes little Nick, they will wise up and bring him back."

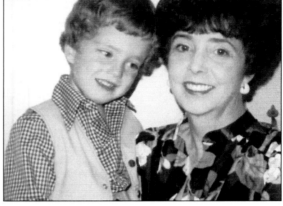

That day came way too early. I was only 12 when my mom passed away. As bad as my memory is today, I remember that night like it was yesterday. I remember my dad and I were having a celebratory conversation out on our deck just a few days before she passed. He was telling me that mom's condition was improving and she was almost "out of the woods."

I remember him saying he was looking forward to bringing her home from the hospital if she kept improving. That is why I will never forget being awoken in the middle of the night a few days later by my dad. I think it was the first time I ever saw him cry. He just hugged me and told me that my mom had died.

You see, my dad was an imposing man at about 6 feet, 1 inch, 275 pounds – most of which was muscle he had built throughout a career as a carpenter and truck driver. He was the kindest, gentlest, most patient man I have ever known. My mom, on the other hand, at about 5-8 and maybe 125 pounds when she was healthy, was the strict disciplinarian.

I was born a very cute, curly haired little boy who often could not pronounce certain sounds of the alphabet. This became a real problem, as my dad was a truck driver and my long-time babysitter's husband and son were named Chuck. So when I told people my dad was a trucker and he had a big truck, it became very comical.

Ironically, my young son Nicholas has the same problem. When he goes to the bank, the teller asks him if he wants a little sucker or a big sucker. He, of course, says he wants a big *ucker! Our family dentist recently scolded Nicholas and told him, "No sucking your thumb!" Nicholas now runs around the house telling family members the dentist said "No *ucking my thumb!" I guess the leaf did not fall far from the tree, as they say.

From the time I was two until I was five, I literally ate only grilled cheese sandwiches. That would explain why all my children like them and they are no longer one of my favorite choices for dinner.

When I was born, I immediately had a guard dog in the form of a Miniature Schnauzer named Woody. Woody was a very old dog, and my family members were afraid there were going to be issues with this dog. My siblings were all older, and Woody had not had a child to compete with for household attention in quite some time. However, Woody and I had an immediate connection. He used to lay under my bassinet and growl harshly if anyone came near it.

I was a very talkative child, but that was probably because I was usually around adults. I knew my two sisters like the back of my hand. If Nancy –16 when I was born – ever wore Nora's clothes, who was 11, or vice versa, I would yell at them. I pretty much grew up with five parents: my mom, my dad and my siblings Jay, Nancy and Nora. Anytime I did something wrong, I got yelled at by all five of them. More importantly, I received a great amount of attention and love from all of them.

My sister Nancy remembers never resenting having me around or having to watch me. She never thought it was odd that her job was to get me ready and take me to the babysitter before going to high school. Her high school friends always laughed at her because she smelled like baby lotion.

I was also known as a little slob, as legend has it. I had a habit of eating in our family den. When I was done, I would shove all the wrappers and garbage under the couch or in the cushions.

As a young boy, my passions were football and baseball cards. When I was twelve, I had over 500,000 cards. The crazy thing was I had the name, position and team of every one of those players memorized. What makes that ironic is now I can barely remember anything unless I write in my planner, save it to my phone, or have a message blinking in neon lights in my cubicle at school. Wow, how the effects of cancer have changed me.

There are a number of skills I have lost due to cancer's effects. I often think if I had some of the memory, focus and concentration abilities I had when I was growing up, my life would be much easier. But a life with a terrible memory, difficulties with concentration and numerous other misgivings is definitely better than no life at all. That I am sure of.

I lived and breathed sports as a young kid. I was ultra-competitive. In high school, I competed in football, basketball, baseball and golf. Athletics was in my blood early on, as it started with neighborhood tackle football and whiffleball games that were more intense than anything. Growing up in a village of 1,400 people, the children just naturally met and played outside all day.

We would leave our homes at 8 in the morning and be outside until lunch. After lunch, we would be gone until dinner. Basically, aside from meals, our summer days were consumed by outside activity. I think it was ultimately that competitiveness and drive that helped me overcome cancer and its many effects. It was also a time where I forged relationships with people who today remain lifelong friends.

My brother, Jay, was 17 when I was born. Needless to say, he did not want anything to do with me. He was annoyed by my existence. I feel like he always felt compelled to maintain this presence as a role model to me. He really felt like he needed to protect me. He always was a bit guarded around me. He wanted me to grow up as a respectful man.

Even with our age discrepancy, we had a balance of a lot in common and a lot of differences. One of the things I remember most was a card he wrote me a few years after I had been sick. He said: "Nick, I know typically it is the little brother who looks up to the big brother, but in our case I wanted you to know how much I look up to you and all that you have been through and accomplished."

That, to this day, is one of best compliments I have ever received. Big brothers typically do not say that to their little brothers. I followed Jay everywhere when I was little. I waited every night until he got home so we could watch TV together. He brought me to all of his softball games and made sure I was the bat boy for every one of them.

We shared an absolute passion for the Green Bay Packers and he introduced me to the Eagles rock band. My junior year in high school, he surprised me with tickets to the Eagles' "Hell Freezes Over" concert at the Bradley Center in Milwaukee. Keep in mind he was 34 years old and had numerous friends he could have taken.

Jay and I sat in section 110, rows one and two, seats ten and eleven at Lambeau Field for over twenty years and made great memories as Green Bay Packers fans. When I was sick, my brother vowed he would never return to a game in those seats without me by his side.

When I was sick in a Chicago hospital, he shaved my face and helped me with other things only a brother can help someone do. We did, however, agree that he not shave my face during football games. We both would be too emotional and it was not a good time to have a blade around.

The day Jay went to buy himself an official Green Bay Packers stock certificate of ownership, I'm sure you can guess who else he bought one for. We owned the Packers together, and we cheered them on together for over twenty years in section 110. More importantly, we loved each other regardless of our age difference. Jay was also my godfather, and I am the godfather of his beautiful daughter, Maureen.

My sister, Nancy, was 16 when I was born. Unlike my brother, she was never embarrassed as a high school student to have a baby brother. In fact, she did not even mind getting me ready in the morning, as most of the time my mom and dad were already gone to work. Nancy routinely dressed me, fed me and dropped me off at the babysitter's before going to school. She was and still is like a second mother to me. When I was young and our mom was very sick, it was very natural for her to play mom in a lot of different ways.

In fact, as my mom got sicker and I got older, it became routine for me to spend most of my summer vacations living with Nancy, her husband, Omar, and their young family. They lived in Southern Wisconsin, and I really enjoyed spending as much time with them as I could. My sister and her husband were blessed to have four great children, two of which happen to have Down syndrome.

Katie is 31 and Max 21 as I write this. Katie was my first niece when I was only eight years old. It is very cool to have a niece when you are in second grade. When she was born, nobody ever came right out and told me she had Down syndrome. I guess I just kind of figured it out at my young age.

I remember pushing her in a shopping cart at Shopko when I was ten and she was two. I remember watching people stare at her the feeling it gave me. That is when I realized Katie was different, but she was special and she was my niece. Ironically, she and Max are the reason I am a special education teacher at Preble High School today.

I experienced those same stares or glares later in my life when I returned after all the grueling surgeries, therapies and treatments from brain cancer. I guess I understand it better today, but at the time it was tearing me apart the way people looked at me. I had lost sixty pounds, sported scars all over my head, and I had a lazy eye and slouched posture from the stroke.

Nobody looked at me like the dean's list student or the football player anymore. They looked at me like I was different; the same way I remember them looking at my niece years ago. It is a bad feeling. Being different than the societal norm is an intimidating place to find yourself. Just like Katie and Max have always had great family support to keep them shielded from any outside criticism, so have I.

They had two brothers to help them. Garret and Joe were right between them in age. Garret is currently a special education teacher and a coach just like me. He and his wife Tara just had their first little boy. Joe just came back from the Army after spending much of the past year on the border of Afghanistan and Pakistan.

My youngest sister, Nora, was eleven when I was born and still jokes about how she was robbed of being the baby of the family. While Nancy was a bit more of a motherly figure, Nora did not like changing diapers or any of the gross tendencies that come with suddenly having a little brother. Nora often jokes that if I am ever diagnosed with diabetes, it is her fault. Apparently, when I was a baby and crying, she would roll my pacifier in sugar and stick it in my mouth. That was a resentful, eleven-year-old's way of dealing with a crabby little brother she had not fully embraced as part of her family.

She did, however, know how to utilize my strengths and talents as a young boy. While she would babysit me, she would talk about how great I was at making banana splits. She would go on and on about how I sliced the bananas and put just the right amount of chocolate syrup on the ice cream. Nora would tell me how only I knew the right amount of nuts to put on the ice cream.

I now know that this was a complete load of baloney. But at the time, it was a clever way to avoid getting off the couch during her favorite show and still enjoy the luxury of a well-made banana split. Everybody won. I got to eat ice cream, too. I guess ice cream just makes everything better in life.

Even though my mom and I never had a typical mother-son relationship, I always knew with her spirit and protection of me, I never really had anything to worry about as long as she was around. I may not have always appreciated her enough, but I never, ever questioned her loyalty and protection of me.

That is why her death turned my world around. She was my caregiver and the person who kept everything afloat in our household. My dad worked long and crazy hours. I saw him very little. The night my dad woke me up to tell me my mom died was horrifying.

Who was going to take care of me? My dad was always gone. My siblings had moved out of the house. There was nobody. My dad had to work. He was still years away from retirement. What was going to happen to me? I had a friend who's mom died, but his siblings were young like him and his dad had a job in which he came home every night. This was not fair.

In the transition period after my mom died, my dad's twin sisters took care of me. While they were amazing women and a great help to my dad, I did not want anything to do with them. They were much older than my dad and neither of them had children of their own. What did they know about a cocky little middle school kid?

Speaking of school, life did not get any better a few months after my mom died and it was time for me to go back to school. My negative behavior at school escalated. Acting out and being the class clown was my way of showing everyone that my mom's death hadn't affected me. While that was wrong of me to do, the discipline procedures I faced at my Catholic grade school were even worse.

I remember sitting in our principal's office when Sister K told me my behaviors were due to my mom's death and the solution was that I needed to cry more. You see, Sister K had not seen me cry, so therefore she did not think I did at all. I'll never forget the time she would not let me leave her office until I actually broke down and cried in front of her. After quite a while, I eventually cried.

I do not think my crying had anything to do with mom's death. At the time, I just wanted to get the hell out of her office and go play football at recess. Believe me, if anything was going to help me with the issues I had after my mom died, it was not going to be artificially crying in some nun's office. My healing process was better suited for a good, old-fashioned football game at recess. That would relieve much more tension.

I was very angry during the period when my two aunts were in charge of me. I was very bitter that my mom was gone and my dad was always working. Little did I know my dad sensed this very early after my mom died. Even though he was grieving more than anyone, he had immediately begun making plans to be there for his youngest son full-time.

My dad realized he needed to retire early from truck driving, find a part-time job and make sure he was there for me. The man I had hardly known and I were now going to be full-time roommates. That decision by my dad was a major sacrifice. But it was one I believe may have saved my life.

From that day on, every decision my dad made had my best interests in mind. That is probably why I began developing a fear that would overwhelm my adolescent and young adult years. As I became closer and closer with my dad, the possibility of losing my only living parent became a fear that consumed my life. I would worry night and day that something was going to happen to my dad. I was so afraid something bad was going to happen and that I was going to be without parents altogether.

I was so scared I was going to be the only kid to graduate from eighth grade with no parents. And then my fear was graduating from high school without any parents. After that, it was would I receive my college degree with no parents at my side? While my siblings all filled some parental roles when I was young, the thought of finishing childhood and adolescence without at least one parent was something that overwhelmed me as a young person.

I developed this superstitious ritual every time I saw my dad or spoke to him, I could not leave him without giving him a hug and telling him "thank you" and "I love you." I never hung up the phone with him without speaking those same words. While it may have seemed a bit over the top to him and others around us at times, I never stopped this ritual for the sixteen years between my mom's death and my dad's death.

Over those years, my dad and I became best friends until the day he died.

Chapter 3

Football and the Green Bay Packers

Growing up, the Green Bay Packers and football in general were synonymous with the Nesvacil family. While our autumn weeks were filled with anticipation for those Packer game days, our hearts were filled with passion for the game. Football was a common ground for everyone in our family, and everyone adored the Packers and their legacy.

This upbringing led me to want to play football in middle school and high school. In high school, I was never the biggest or strongest player on our team, but I was a two-way starter who played with a passion others did not have. While I was a decent player during those prep years, no one had college football on their radar for me. That was, no one except me.

I was bound and determined to keep my football career going after high school. Even after my high school coach told me I was probably too small and too slow, I was sure I was capable of playing at the next level. I had been an all-conference player in high school. While I respected my football coach greatly, I did not agree with him when he told me I could not

play football at St. Norbert
College, a liberal arts college in
De Pere, Wisconsin, just outside
Green Bay.

It was October 1994 and
an amazingly beautiful fall day.
There was a slight breeze
blowing through the colored
trees surrounding St. Norbert's
old Minahan Stadium. The smell
of autumn, mixed with the
ability for me to play the game I
so dearly loved, made this day
seemingly perfect.

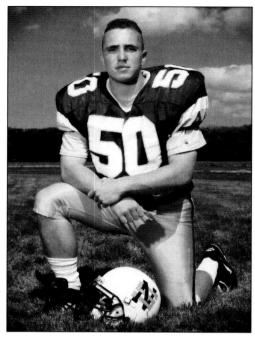

A familiar feeling of adrenaline coursed through my veins as I
prepared to snap the football. I was the center. The man across from me was
my opponent, the other team's nose-tackle. I was 220 pounds and he was 315
pounds.

For most of the game, we had battled evenly. Everything came down
to this key fourth down and goal to go. As I snapped the ball, I knew
immediately I had great leverage on my opponent and there was no way I
was going to lose on this particular play.

I drove this mammoth human being back as if he was on roller skates,
giving me a feeling of total domination. That is, until I felt as though
someone had shot a bullet into my left knee. The instantaneous pain running
through my leg was excruciating. It was the worse pain I had ever felt at that

point of my life. The next thing I remember was someone saying, "We are going to need an ambulance."

Football is a game in which the offense gets four downs, or opportunities, to reach their short-term goal of a first down. In most cases, the offense also has a more long-term goal of scoring a touchdown, which it can achieve in a variety of ways.

My life has sort of been broken down into four downs – just like a football team's offense. First down for me was realizing the harsh reality that after seven years of lining up and playing football every fall, my career was likely over after having my right kneecap shattered like a car windshield hit by a wrecking ball.

This was it. No more football is what most people told me. I did not want to buy that opinion. Even though the chances of a full recovery and return to the gridiron were unlikely, I was not ready to give up the game I love. I spent months in physical therapy with a therapist who was bigger and louder than any football coach I had ever had.

Her name was Michelle, and my days with her were hell. I used to say, "Off to hell with Michelle!" After about six weeks of therapy with Michelle, I began rehabbing on my own in our college weight room at Schuldes Sports Center.

This was difficult. While I was conditioning one body part that had once resembled a very strong and powerful leg, I had to sit and watch all these other college athletes building their muscle and cardiovascular systems to be better prepared for the big game or a championship race. My only goal was to get off the crutches that had been with me for almost two and a half months.

Needless to say, if this knee injury was first down in my life, I had been tackled for a big loss and was facing second and long on the next down. Little did I know how long of a challenge I would face on the second big down of my life.

The days of rehabbing in the sports center became long and depressing for a young guy who just wanted to run out on the football field and tackle someone (preferably the guy who decided to stick his helmet into my kneecap). The rehabbing, along with the stress of finals in the spring of 1995, really had me at one of my lowest points.

All this stress in my life had caused me to have headaches that seemed to get a little worse each day. They were accompanied by overall body aches and blurry vision. I guess rehabbing your broken leg during the day and pulling late-night study sessions would cause these types of repercussions.

All these physical symptoms at least were making my shattered kneecap the lesser of two evils – for the time being. Soon, however, I found out my kneecap would only be a distant afterthought when it came to second down and long.

As the kneecap slowly made progress, my headaches and blurry vision seemed to intensify. They intensified by the day, if not the hour. After engaging in a lot of self-talk and unsolicited bargaining, I realized something more than my injury and finals was going on. In a matter of days, my girlfriend and I visited an optometrist and then an ophthalmologist. The news was good. Nothing was wrong with my eyes.

But the news was also bad. The second eye doctor recommended I see a neurologist very soon. All I knew about neurology was that it had something to do with the brain. That scared me a lot.

I had that same feeling I had on first down when I hurt my knee. Now, however, there was much more of the unknown. We were not talking about a shattered kneecap, but the possibility of a problem with my brain. I thought first down and a knee injury put me in a long-yardage, desperate-type of situation.

I had no idea what I was up against next. It was going to be the second down of a lifetime. The biggest challenge of my life.

Throughout my football career, there was only one time the word "quit" had come into my mind. I was fifteen and a freshman in high school. I had just finished up a scrimmage in which I played very poorly. After the scrimmage, my coach told me I was being replaced as the starting offensive tackle. I was devastated. I was pissed off. I wanted nothing to with my coach or team or the game of football.

I went home to express my opinions to my dad about how angry I was. My dad looked at me and said, "People in this family do not quit." He said, "Go back to practice, work your butt off and get back into the starting lineup."

Do you think blocking a 300-pound, all-conference player in high school is scary?

Do you think shattering your kneecap in a college football game is scary?

Do you think the idea of not ever being able to play football again is scary?

I thought they were at the time. Little did I know how relatively minor those issues were compared to what I was about to face. Scary took on a whole new meaning when I heard those three words: "You have cancer."

One minute you're living life to the fullest, and the next, three words slam you and your life face-down in the dirt.

Cancer's like that. This disease, this horrible, confounding disease, takes people. It takes good, strong people. It takes them and it pushes them – hard. It pushes them down – it pushes them into the dirt.

Despite strong will, despite dynamic personalities and all the optimism in the world, this disease pushes ... and pushes ... and pushes. It pushes hundreds of thousands of people a day. It pushes millions of people a year. It pushes them. Facedown down in the dirt. Then it pounds them down. Again, again, and again. Just try to get up. Just try.

I thought I had experienced fear a time or two in my life. I had no idea what fear was until I was the "you" in the "You have cancer" statement.

I'm an athlete, but I've never thrown a javelin. Now I felt that disease pierce my heart, my hopes, and my life like a javelin. I had never been slammed this hard in all of my toughest football games. Yeah, I've had the wind knocked out of me. But I always got up. I always got up to get back in the game.

But cancer? That's a different game with different rules. This game was being played with me. With my life.

Why? Why me? Why me?

You know how your body gets all charged-up for a game? The adrenalin. That feeling. The feeling like you can't be beat. The adrenalin's flowing. Well, cancer takes that feeling. It steals that adrenalin and it turns it against you. The disease knows how athletic you are and it steals that ability. Cancer steals and it keeps stealing until there's nothing left.

Once I had heard those three words, the sensation began to control me. My body became desperate. I was afraid to breathe. I wanted to kill the monster inside of me and get my life back to normal. All I wanted was the life I had twenty-four hours ago. Now, cancer had my life. This was no game. This was serious.

Yet, in many ways, this competition of me versus cancer would be the biggest competition of my life. I hadn't trained for this one and I didn't know the rules. According to my doctors, we were already at halftime and I was losing. I was losing fast.

In the cancer game, everything gets prioritized differently. Acceptance on a college campus or poor preparation on a philosophy exam are not things to fear. They were simply minor scares. Finding out you have a big game with cancer is humbling and humanizing.

I couldn't verbalize scared, but I knew what it felt like. Another battle that pulsed through my veins was the constant self-talk. Even when I didn't realize it, I constantly entertained an internal dialogue. I was arguing with my body – yes, arguing. Isn't that crazy? Isn't that stupid? No athlete lets that kind of fear take over. But I did.

I was training for a new game. I had to condition myself, and the first series of exercises I had to repeat over and over again was to control that self-talk. If I didn't, it would eat me alive, just like those cancer cells that were devouring me every minute of every day.

My cancer was brain cancer. I kept thinking of those science fiction shows where the brain gets rewired and destroys the character's body. But this was no sci-fi show. This was the real thing.

But I had that feeling. I had that caution. I had that constant, nagging fear. "Don't let the cancer take over MY brain. It's mine. My life is mine. I have to fight. And keep fighting. And keep fighting."

So I was thrown onto the field for the biggest game of my life. For years and years, I had been coached to be prepared, to be in shape, to have concentration and control. That focus now was under attack twenty-four hours a day. When I talked to people, I talked to myself. When I went through my daily routine, I talked to myself. Even when I dreamed, I talked to myself. That voice of cancer was always there. I tried to separate the two: what's really coming from my brain and what's really coming from the cancer?

This is what scared feels like: "Why me? What are my chances? Hey, maybe someone can help me out of this. I might wake up. I've had dreams like this before. I need to wake up. I just need to wake up."

But I'm here, and I have cancer. "I need to wake up. But I'm dying. How soon? Do I tell everyone? Cancer picked me. It knows I'm tough. I can beat it. Cancer's beating me. I'm scared. I'm the honors student. I'm the good kid. I'm on the football team. I was on the football team. Didn't I prove myself in college? Didn't I show I was good? Didn't I show I was strong? Why am I being punished?"

My outward optimism wasn't really optimism at all. It was a façade. I didn't want people to know about that battle inside of me. I hated it that people now saw me, Nick, the poor guy with cancer. Poor Nick.

I think my schooling and training instinctively made me rationalize my situation. It was grim, but I had licked every other challenge I faced in my life. It was basically this: Nick versus cancer. That's all it was. Nick versus cancer. It was now definitely fourth down and long.

Who would win? Who would die? That was the dark, cold mystery that dampened my spirits. If I lived, I knew this experience was going to change my life forever.

After being injured and realizing my future in football was not going to be as a player, I knew my passion for the game was still strong, as was my passion for my favorite NFL team, the Green Bay Packers.

I was hooked on the Packers at an early age. I remember how bad the Packers were throughout the 1980s. It never fazed me, as I was born into a tradition of hard-core Packer fans regardless of their lack of success. I remember my grade school buddies and how they all fell in love with other teams. They all jumped on the bandwagons of the Oakland Raiders, Dallas Cowboys and in some cases even the rival Chicago Bears.

Not me. The Packers were my one and only team from day one. It's been a love affair that has never wavered. My dad took me to my first game when I was eight years old. I will never forget it. If I wasn't completely a Packers addict before that, walking into Lambeau Field for the first time was the absolute clincher.

From that point, I have only missed a handful of Packers home games in more than three decades. Either as a season ticket holder or as employee of the Packers, I have seen every momentous moment the organization has experienced since then.

Returning to St. Norbert College during my recovery, I was a lost soul, searching for some semblance of my former self. I longed to be part of something other than my cancer recovery. I wanted to be part of something like the Green Bay Packers. I had remembered meeting the legendary Lee Remmel when I was a young boy. Lee was a man who knew more about the Packers than anyone I knew. Aside from being the Packers' director of public relations and later the team's official historian, he had also covered the team for the local newspaper for many years.

The fall after my illness, I decided I was going to call Lee and inquire about any employment opportunities in the Packers' public relations department. He granted me a meeting and we spent over an hour together. I spoke of my passion for the Packers and of my recent struggles with my health.

He confided with me that he, too, had gone through a brain tumor when he was young. While his memory of that period was a bit sketchy, we began bonding more about some of the amazing stories he was telling me about Packers history.

I remember this amazing man telling me stories about Vince Lombardi arriving in Green Bay to take over the Packers' head coaching duties in 1959, and how at one point, Don Shula almost became the Packers' head coach. Shula went on to win two Super Bowls as coach of the Miami Dolphins and holds the record for most coaching victories in NFL history. Sitting with Lee that day was one of my life highlights.

What made the conversation so great was that he offered me a game day position working as a public relations intern during home games at Lambeau Field. I spent game days working in the auxiliary press box. My job was simply to maintain professionalism among the many field scouts from the other NFL teams and public relations people from the visiting team.

While this internship was small and truly had to be begged for, it ended up being another step back to normality, giving me a true sense of accomplishment. Feeling like I was a small part of the organization that I loved since I was five-years old made me feel like I had achieved something. This was a big deal. I had a parking pass, a jacket and tie, and another reason to think I was going to make it all the way back.

I worked on home game days for the Packers for two seasons. In the second season, I even helped out in the Lambeau Field offices one day per week. While the Packers could have easily made it without me there, I do not know what I would have done without something like that to hold onto.

It was a great experience and just what I needed at the time. I also had the opportunity to work under one of the true Packers legends in Lee Remmel, who devoted his entire life to working closely with the organization. A great man.

When I was sick and in the hospital in Green Bay, I received a visit from legendary Packers center Larry McCarren. Larry is now the voice of the Packers on the radio and is widely known throughout Wisconsin for his affiliation with the team.

Larry was a sportscaster with one of the local TV stations when I was in high school, and he had a segment once a week called "Challenge the Rock." Rock was Larry's nickname from his playing days at the University of Illinois and with the Packers. Each week on the show, someone from the community would challenge him at one of their unique talents.

I developed a unique talent as a basketball player at Denmark High School. As a player who did not see an abundance of playing time, I loved basketball for what it was: a competitive sport where I was able to let off steam and be with my friends. I did not love it like football, but it was great being part of a team and competing. Not being overly serious about my future in basketball, I developed a unique skill in my time around the court. Believe it or not, I could shoot a basketball through the hoop with incredible consistency from half court while sitting down.

Unbeknownst to me, one day I was called down to the office and told to report to the gymnasium. When I walked in, there were about a hundred students and all my closest friends. On top of that, Larry McCarren and his TV crew were there to film that week's version of "Challenge the Rock." My friends had secretly called Larry and told him of my unique skill. He had to see it to believe it. Everyone was there to witness me challenge him.

I made the half-court shot sitting down and Larry did not even get close. My friends cheered loudly. It was a great experience. I remember Larry leading off the sports coverage during the 6:00 news saying, "Nick Nesvacil is an all-conference football player at Denmark High School, and he ain't bad at basketball, either."

Having Larry stop by the hospital that day to check on me and wish me the best meant the world to me. To this day, I see Larry at church and in the community and he always thanks me for what STINGCANCER has done in the Green Bay community. He is a great man and a great representation of what Green Bay and the Packers are all about.

Even when I moved from a Green Bay hospital to a Chicago hospital, I still received amazing support from the Packers. I'll never forget one early morning I was lying in my hospital bed talking to my dad and brother. The phone rang, and a man with a very deep, hoarse voice said, "Hello, is this Nick Nesvacil?" I replied yes. The voice sounded very familiar, but it couldn't be who I was thinking it was. Could it?

He said, "Nick, this is Reggie White of the Packers."

When I said, "Hello, Reggie," I will never forget how fast my dad and brother's heads whipped away from the television. You see, we only knew one Reggie, and that was the one who played on the defensive line for the Packers. Reggie White! The Minister of Defense! One of best players in NFL history! The guy who teamed with Brett Favre to bring the Packers back to prominence!

We spoke for a few minutes about what I was going through. I remember thinking it was training camp and I could hear players in the background. I knew Reggie must have been calling from the locker room in between practices.

Before hanging up, Reggie kindly asked if we could say a prayer together. Talk about motivation to get better! Aside from a great group of family and friends, my support group now included the all-time NFL leader in sacks at the time.

My support list also includes Jerry Parins. Jerry was a long-time Green Bay police officer and later director of security for the Green Bay Packers. He's also a cancer survivor and someone who has become an invaluable friend to me.

About eight years ago, STINGCANCER was highlighted in our local newspaper. A day later, I received a phone call from Jerry and a request to meet with him at his office in Lambeau Field. Of course, I jumped at this opportunity. At the time, I was thirty years old and Jerry was sixty-four. Age could not separate all Jerry and I had in common. There was much more than an allegiance to the great city of Green Bay and a passion for the Packers we shared. We were both absolutely dedicated to the fight against cancer.

What Jerry was doing to battle cancer with the help of the Packers organization, I was doing the same through the support of Preble High School and the Green Bay Area Public School District.

Jerry and I had an instant connection. We shared a passion against cancer that could not be challenged. We talked Packers, cancer and about "giving back" that day.

Jerry holds an annual "Cruise for Cancer" event in which he and hundreds of his friends ride their motorcycles to raise money. Jerry disperses the money raised back into the Green Bay community, primarily for health-care purposes.

That day in Jerry's office he asked me if I would be an honorary guest on his ride. Of course I accepted, and was honored to be part of this amazing day. My family and I were driven by Pepper Burruss, the long-time Packers trainer. I was also presented with a Packers jersey with the number 30 on it, signifying my age at the time. Jerry later had that jersey autographed by Packers greats Brett Favre and Ahman Green.

Jerry annually visits STINGCANCER meetings and helps educate our students about cancer. He also graciously donates money to our cause. He has gone so far over the years to have Brett and Deanna Favre autograph STINGCANCER hats and t-shirts.

Even though Jerry has dined with stars, rubbed elbows with Pro Football Hall of Famers and taken pictures with presidents, he is one of the most humble and gracious men I have ever known. I look at Jerry as a father figure, as he has given me so much advice and inspiration over the years.

I continue to spend my summers and falls working as a part-time employee in the Packers Pro Shop, the team's retail store. While it is only a seasonal position, it allows me to be a small part of an organization that has done so much for me. I get to meet amazing people from all over the world who have a strong passion for the Packers.

I remember when I was a patient in Chicago, there was one nurse who was a die-hard Packers fan. She was obviously in the minority in a Chicago hospital. However, she would sneak in and talk Packers with me. It always made me feel closer to home. She made me realize then the power of being a Packers fan and how it truly brings people together.

I have seen that phenomenon on display again and again as an employee in the Packers Pro Shop. I have met so many people from across the globe who have the same passion for the team that I have. Also, many of them have stories about how the Packers organization helped them during some of their darkest hours.

The Packers are a large reason why Northeast Wisconsin is a great place to live. It is also a wonderful area where people are about giving love and support to those in need. I found that somebody's always got your back if you live in the Green Bay area.

Also, for the last five years, the Packers organization has supported STINGCANCER by allowing their employees to wear yellow on STINGCANCER's annual Wear Yellow Day in May. They purchase shirts for their employees and celebrate the fight against cancer along with the rest of the area. The Packers are truly a great supporter of those in need throughout Northeast Wisconsin. They are much more than just a football team.

Chapter 4

My Dad

My dad was and always will be my best friend. Growing up, I did not know this hardworking truck driver who worked long days and nights and was not always readily available to my childhood needs. I always respected him for how hard he worked, but I did not know him all that well. That was until I was twelve years old and my mom died of Crohn's disease.

With my older siblings already moved out of our house, my dad had only one option. It was to retire early, take on a part time job and take care of me full time. Over the next twelve years, he exceeded any expectations of any father on the planet. He and I become much more than father and son. He was much more to me. He was my dad. He was my big brother. He was my shoulder to lean on. He was my roommate. Most of all, he was my best friend. And in June of 1996, I quickly found out I needed a best friend more than ever.

When I was diagnosed with cancer, my dad never batted an eye – at least not in front of his son who was scared out of his mind. He simply gathered the people who were closest to us, told them that nobody was going to quit in the fight against this cancer, and that come hell or high water, we were not going to let cancer take our youngest family member.

My dad, Nic Nesvacil, was a very strong man. He was the youngest of four siblings and veteran of the Korean War. Ten years after watching the love of his life die, he was not about to watch his youngest son fall victim to the same fate because of cancer. My dad was there for every appointment, check-up, surgery and everything else I needed. He continuously got me out of bed when I could not get myself out to go to a treatment.

He never outwardly showed any sign of weakness or quit when it came to me and this horrible disease. Whether or not it was always genuine, I do not know. But I do know, because he always displayed a brave front, that I never believed I would die with him by my side. He was a quiet man with a sense of humor and a passion for his family.

My dad always instilled confidence in me when I needed it most. When I decided to play football at St. Norbert College after high school, I encountered some pushback from my high school coach. He said that although I had made all-conference my senior year, he thought I was too small and a bit too slow. When I told my dad what my coach told me, he simply said he knew I could do it if it was something I really wanted to do.

I remember like it was yesterday when I decided I wanted to ask my girlfriend, Maureen, to get married. I was so nervous when I went home to tell my dad of my plans. I remember walking into the kitchen where I grew up. He was sitting at the table reading the paper. I grabbed another section of the paper and sat at the other end of our long kitchen table. After fidgeting around for about five minutes, I finally got the courage up to tell him that I needed to ask him something.

No sooner could I say, "Dad, I need to ask you a question," that he immediately replied back, "Ask her to marry you, she's a beautiful girl." It was like he knew my every move.

And this all happened when he was very sick and for the most part homebound. Throughout my illness and later my dad's health struggles, we grew to know each other on a level in which few fathers and sons probably ever reach. I am very proud of that.

Whenever he helped out my siblings in any way, he always made sure that the rest of my siblings received equal benefits. For example, when I went on spring break, he gave me $100. He then made sure each of my siblings knew what he did and he gave them each the same. He was the fairest person I have ever known. I do think whether he would admit it or not, he gave me a gift that nobody else in our family received. He gave me the gift of strength when I needed it most. He gave me the gift of perseverance when the obstacles of football or cancer or whatever life threw at me seemed insurmountable. He gave me survival, as he never had a doubt I was going to survive cancer and all of its effects.

He is the main reason why I am here today. He gave me the gift of life. Not only did he refuse to let cancer kill me, he also showed me how to live life. Today, I am the husband I am because of my dad; the father I am because of my dad; the teacher I am because of my dad. Today, I am the leader I am because of my dad. Throughout the months and years of chemotherapy, radiation, speech therapy, occupational therapy and physical therapy, I know he was as mentally exhausted as I was. But never once did he show any sort of weakness or negativity.

He was truly my rock. Ironically, seven years later, our roles were reversed. My dad was now the one diagnosed with colon cancer.

Unfortunately, because of some unhealthy choices and the advanced stage of his cancer, I was unable to help my dad the way he helped me. But I can say that every day when I wake up, I thank God for my dad and pray to God that I can be half the dad to my kids that he was to me.

When I was sick, my support group was led by the strongest man I have ever known. Ironically, he was taken by cancer just seven short years after he helped me overcome it. People typically look at their fathers as disciplinarians, role models or simply the man who lives in their house and makes most of the rules.

My dad was different. He was the single parent and my roommate for thirteen years after my mom died. He was my mom and my dad. He was my roommate and my dad. He definitely was my role model. He was my dad. He most certainly was my mentor. He was my dad. He was my rock. He was my dad. He was and always will be my best friend. He was and always will be my dad.

I can wholeheartedly say that without my dad, I would not be here today. When he found out his twenty-year-old son had brain cancer, he never batted an eye. He gathered my family together and immediately instilled the confidence in them that they would need in order to prepare themselves for what our family was about to go through. I knew then that my dad was going to make sure somehow, some way, I was not going to die. Not on his watch!

No matter how grim things may have looked or how negative the endless doctors' reports got, my dad always looked at our battle as one we were going to win. Whether it was sitting at my bedside for hours on end in the hospital, dragging me out of bed and into the car for another chemo treatment or patting my back while I was throwing up after a radiation appointment, my dad never flinched.

We were going to win this hellish battle as a family. That was all there was to it. I think my brother, Jay, summed it up nicely when he said that my dad was a pillar of strength. My sister-in-law, Theresa, vividly remembers an example of my dad's strength. She said, "Nick, the thing that stands out the most during your experience with cancer in the summer of 1996 was when you were going to undergo your major brain tumor surgery at Children's Hospital in Chicago. The doctors' assistants were ready to take you in, and it was our time to say goodbye.

"Of course, for all of us, this was an extremely difficult time. Your dad was first. And I think Jay and I were last. I can remember standing in line thinking, 'What can I say to this kid to comfort, to support him or even if I should say goodbye?' We all knew – good or bad – that this would be a life-changing surgery for you. I know we were all saying silent prayers for you. Making deals with God. At least I know that is what I was doing.

"Your dad was the first one to address you. I can remember just when you think you do not have the strength to hide how scared you are for your brother-in-law, someone like your father stands up and shows his undeniable faith, love and belief in you. He truly believed at that time you would come out of this okay. I'll never forget it.

"He took you by your hand, kissed your forehead and said, 'Be strong, my son, be strong.' He walked away, and the rest of us followed his lead. I look back at that moment, and after having kids, I now realize how strong of a man your dad was. Your dad knew you were in for the battle of your life. And yet, he somehow knew you were going to walk away from this. It was the best example of faith I've seen in my entire life."

When I finally was getting prepared to graduate from St. Norbert, I remember talking to my dad. He told me I should get a graduation ring. I had never thought about it much. After his suggestion, I explored the possibility only to find the prices to be way too high for my dad to afford. I left the magazine in which we looked at college rings somewhere at my dad's house and honestly never gave it another thought.

I would have loved a ring, but the mere fact that my dad had even brought up the idea of purchasing one meant a lot to me. I knew because of all the medical bills and doing everything in his power to keep his son alive, he 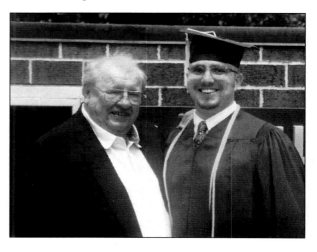 was experiencing a financial strain. That is why after leaving the magazine at my dad's house, I forgot about it.

That was until a few days before my college graduation when he gave me an amazing gold ring that was highlighted with my area of study, the year I graduated and a gold football in the middle of the green diamond. I was totally overwhelmed. I told him he should not have done such a thing.

While I immediately fell in love with the ring, I knew that the cost of it was not in my dad's current price range. My dad's response was that after everything I had been through, I must have been crazy to think he wasn't going to give me the ring I deserved. He said it was a perfect symbol for everything I had overcome to receive my diploma and graduate with honors.

Chapter 5

The Value of Friends

There is no doubt in my mind that my family and friends gave me the hope and will to stay alive. Like all of God's creatures, human beings have a fierce instinct for survival: the will to live. That instinct to not give up at any cost is a natural impulse in all of us. Yet, mental and physical effects of disease easily destroy some people, while others call on inner resources to get them through the experience.

Where does that inner strength come from? Maybe the survivors have learned to be resilient by getting through all that they have. Getting stronger, tougher and more confident in the process. Maybe the small flame of determination that makes us shine brightest in the most difficult times just is not the same with all people.

I believe your flame is lit – in large part – by the support group around you. Aside from my own experience, I believe those who have hope definitely have a major advantage. Could it be that an individual's flame can be strengthened by the support they feel from those closest to them? I believe that is why I am alive to write this book.

Aaron was a 16-year-old baseball player who was an all-city shortstop in Chicago. When I arrived in Chicago at Children's Hospital, I realized I had a roommate I would never forget. I do not remember a lot about Aaron other than his side of the room was filled with trophies, plaques and many other accolades having to do with his baseball prowess.

He seemed like a nice kid. Both of us were fighting brain cancer and I do not remember a lot of our conversations. One thing I do remember hearing is Aaron had a pretty good chance of survival.

His future appeared a lot brighter than mine, as shortly after meeting him I was told I had a meningitis infection and had suffered a stroke back in Green Bay during my initial surgery. I also remember every morning being wheeled out of my room for physical, occupational and speech therapy.

I distinctly remember returning to my room one Saturday morning. Aaron was not there. I guess I assumed he was in therapy, having an updated MRI or receiving some other services. I was informed later in the day of the truth: Aaron's bright prognosis had turned bleak in a hurry.

He had acquired some sort of infection and was now in the ICU. The next evening, my family told me he had died. This absolutely shocked me and sent my confidence reeling.

The interesting thing was that although Aaron had a much more positive prognosis than I did, there was definitely something missing. While my side of the room in that Chicago hospital was always filled with family and friends, his side of the room had visitors only sparingly. Now I do not know Aaron's family demographics or how many friends he had, but it sure seemed like a nice kid like him should have had the same support I did.

According to "Everyone's Guide to Cancer Therapy," doctors have seen how two patients with similar ages, the same diagnosis and degree of illness, and the same treatment program, experience vastly different results. The only noticeable difference between the two was that one person was pessimistic and the other was optimistic.

Just like great support from friends and family can lift one up to new heights, I'm sure it can work in reverse, too. I can't imagine sitting in a hospital room with brain cancer and feeling alone. I never came close to that with all my family and friends at my side throughout my entire journey.

As long as your family, friends and support team can keep a positive attitude, hope can see you through any crisis and times of extreme heartache. Hope, courage, effort, determination, endurance, love and faith all nurture the will to live. All of these are enhanced dramatically by the support of family and friends. However, the road back to health remains a major challenge, even with all the support.

During my sickness, I quickly learned how society values those who can assimilate quickly and bounce back from tragedy without skipping a beat. That's great in theory, but the reality is once cancer has touched your life, nothing will ever be the same.

Relationships are tested and priorities are re-evaluated. Perhaps the most important factor is a survivor has faced mortality and emerged transformed, keenly aware of how fragile life is. Survivors and those close to them must acknowledge all that has happened. It is only then they can move forward and derive meaning from their experience. This is the challenge facing all survivors. With the help of family, friends and a great support group, having cancer can change your life in a positive way.

While counselors and other professionals are very helpful and much needed, I believe close friends are truly the unsung heroes of one's cancer journey. Friends will offer specific help to you. Friends know who you are and what is going to make you feel better.

Friends will respect your care decisions. Friends will help you take your mind off cancer. Friends will value your wishes and understand your character quirks. Friends know you so well they will always bring just the right gifts to put a smile on your face. And most important, true friends won't disappear during the roughest times.

Friends and family are the most important part of your recovery. All the medicine and treatments in the world can't add up to a great network of friends. Counselors and caretakers do a great job in helping you. But for them it is just that, a job. Nothing can stack up against a friend being by your side just because they are your friend. Not even cancer.

My experience has not only changed my views on life, it also has pushed those people closest to me to value life in a stronger way.

While the idea of cancer is never completely gone, neither is the need for special friends. After losing over sixty-five pounds, living with a bald, scarred head and now having a lazy eye, I thought the prospects of someone ever wanting anything to do with me were pretty slim.

On top of those issues, I actually had a hole about the size of a nickel in the back of my head. Even the best baseball cap could not cover up what an ugly duckling I had turned into. When I looked into the mirror, I saw a fragment of my former self.

I could not believe how much my physical appearance had been ravaged over the last year. However, when I met a beautiful girl from St. Norbert College, she obviously saw something different. She saw through the physical, emotional and psychological scars I had.

Maureen Dermody and I became fast friends. Our first date was at Titletown Brewing Company in Green Bay, a cool restaurant in a historic railroad depot. In our initial conversation that night, it came up that both of us had longed to name our first-born daughter Grace. Neither of us knew that we would actually have the opportunity to fulfill our dreams of someday having a daughter with that name.

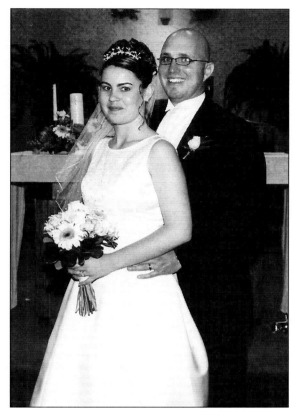

And we sure did not know on that first date we would eventually be married. As our relationship developed, there were a lot of things we were unsure about. That is why I give Maureen so much credit. She is a beautiful girl – both on the inside and out – and could have picked any guy she wanted. Any guy who would have come with a lot less baggage than me.

When I met Maureen, I did not know if I was going to survive. I did not know if I could ever have children after the aggressive chemotherapy and radiation I had been put through. We started on a journey where there were no guarantees for either of us.

Actually, there was one: my assurance that I loved her more than anything. She was also able to tell me she loved me more than anything. It may sound like a fairytale, but sometimes I guess love is truly all you need.

Even though I was unsure of my health moving forward, and my surgical stroke had left me with a terrible memory and concentration issues, Maureen stayed by my side. Even though I told her with all the exhaustive cancer treatments I had been through that children were unlikely in my future, she stayed by my side. I was so nervous to tell her I most likely was not going to be able to father children.

I remember going for a walk around her parents' neighborhood in Milwaukee. My plan was to tell her that night. Maureen, being a first grade teacher and absolutely amazing with any child she encountered, would not respond well to being told children were not an option in our future. I feared that during that walk around the block, we might be having a discussion that would end our relationship.

I was so nervous that I remember realizing we were almost back to her parents' house and I had not gotten up the nerve to tell her yet. What if cancer was going to strike again? My head was swimming. Finally, I just could not take it anymore. I blurted everything out, concluding that I understood if she did not want to continue this relationship.

She looked at me and told me she loved me. She gave me a hug. She simply said, "We can always adopt. I love you more than anything, Nick." That was probably the greatest display of unconditional love I have ever experienced in my life.

After taking so long to tell her and building up so much anxiety, I suddenly felt like the weight of the world had been lifted off my back.

Cancer may be able to beat a lot of things, but it was not going to get the best of the love Maureen and I shared for one another.

Ironically, Maureen and I have had no trouble having children since our marriage in 2003. Rather, it has been unusually easy! It would seem that some miracles just cannot be explained.

I know there are thousands of people out there who have difficulty having children. I do not want to be insensitive to anyone. But for some odd reason it was as if all the radiation and chemotherapy that had ravaged my body had also super-intensified my ability to procreate. Today, we have three beautiful daughters and an incredibly busy son.

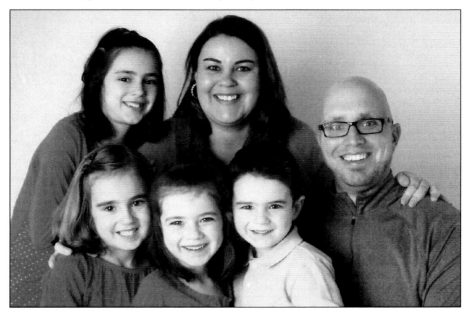

As of this writing, Grace is nine, Claire is seven, Evelyn is five, and Nicholas is four. We call them our four little miracles.

On another note, Maureen and I still go through the normal things all cancer survivors and the people closest to them go through. In our case, we have to deal with my memory and concentration issues almost every day. No matter how much neuropsychology and brain retraining I went through, my mind is nowhere near as sharp as it was before my brain cancer.

After doing some research the last few years, I have realized the amount of stress my brain has gone through is truly amazing. I have found so many of the things I have gone through can and do have long-term effects on memory and the ability to focus and concentrate. Furthermore, in most of the cases I have read about, there is very little that medicine and any type of brain retraining can do. I recently read where a pineal tumor, which is what I had, can have major effects on memory and concentration. I have found that extensive anesthesia can have tons of long-term effects on a person. I have been put to sleep for surgery at least eleven times that I can remember.

I also read how there is tons of evidence that chemotherapy causes long-term memory loss and inability to concentrate, among its many side effects. I underwent some of the most aggressive chemo known to man when I was fighting for my life. Also, the effects of brain radiation are countless and include a lot of evidence of memory and focusing problems.

This adds to the obvious effects that a stroke has on memory. The information about this is extremely grim to read. All these things that have been part of my battle and recovery have had a significant effect on me. I have not even looked into what effect the hundreds of medications and physical trauma of multiple brain surgeries can add to memory loss and inability to focus.

While I recognize my weaknesses in these areas often puts a lot of stress on our relationship and on Maureen especially, I also know that any women who marries a guy who had a hole in his head on their first date is not easily scared off.

Maureen was not part of my life when I was fighting cancer, but she is a major reason why I can proudly call myself a survivor. Much like my dad did when I was battling brain cancer, Maureen refuses to ever let me quit or take the easy way out of something. She is my best friend and the love of my life.

One thing I learned early on with my cancer is you can sit and feel sorry for yourself as long as you want, but you won't see any positive results from doing that, no matter how terrible I felt because of my appearance.

I learned quickly that if I did not change my inward feelings about myself, I was going to be unable to change my outward actions to others. I needed to embrace all the love and support my friends and family were bestowing upon me. Thank God they all loved me enough to keep pushing me to survive and never, ever let me believe I was going to die.

If I was going to survive cancer, I needed to have all my friends and family in my corner. Feeling sorry for myself was not an option. It's like when you're playing cards. The players must accept the cards dealt to them, but ultimately, they choose how to play the hand. Even though the hand dealt to me sucked, I was lucky enough to have a support team that refused to lose. When the opponent is cancer, no one can win the battle alone. So far, my legacy has been as a survivor who knows cancer is the ultimate challenge each and every day.

Attitude is so important in the battle with cancer. It is the difference in one person with cancer thriving and another giving up. There is an old saying I really like: "I cannot always choose what happens to me, but I can always choose what happens in me."

It goes back to what I mentioned regarding that turning point in my life as a freshman football player: my dad said we do not quit in this family.

He basically was telling me that while I could not choose what happened to me on the football field, I could make a choice about how to handle the situation and get myself back in the starting lineup.

Cancer happened to me. *I got cancer, but cancer didn't get me!* It comes down to while we may not have the best of everything, we need to do what we can to make the best of everything.

My friend Darren and I have always been ultra-competitive. He moved

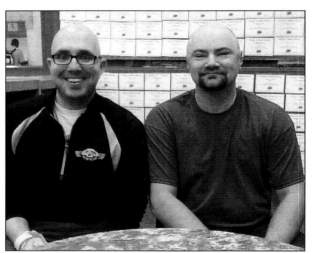

into my neighborhood when we were twelve. Whether it was playing sports or getting up the nerve to ask a girl out, whoever could do it better was the top dog in our neighborhood.

Here are Darren's recollections of our friendship:

"Nick and I became friends when I moved to his neighborhood in 1989. We were in the same grade, but I went to public school and he went to a private school. Shortly after moving in, Nick and I became friends, and he has been my best friend ever since then. Through high school, college, wives and kids.

"I remember the day that Nick said he went to the eye doctor because his vision had changed. That night we played softball against each other in Denmark. I was the leadoff hitter, and on the first pitch of the game I hit a line drive right past Nick's head. When I got to first base, he told me he never saw the ball go by him. Hearing that scared me, and I am sure it scared him as well. Shortly after that, Nick went back to the doctor, and after some tests, he found out he had a brain tumor and it was malignant. That was devastating news to hear when we were so young.

"On the day Nick had his first surgery, I went to the hospital to see him. That was a hard thing to do, not knowing if the doctors would be able to remove the entire tumor. From that day on, I tried to get to the hospital whenever I could. I would go there right after work and stay as long as I could.

"I knew I couldn't do anything medically, but hopefully just sitting by his bed, even if he wasn't awake, it would in some way help him to fight the cancer. I also became closer to his family. In some way, they feel like family to me. After seeing them so much and praying for the same goal, for Nick to get better, it is easy to feel closer to them than just my best friend's family.

"After all of the days Nick spent in the hospital, the day he left St. Vincent, he and I – along with our friend, Francis – went to Kimberly to the World Fastpitch Softball Tournament. We didn't go there to see softball; we went there to spend time with each other and to celebrate finally being out of the hospital.

"And now, eighteen years later, Nick is not the same person he was before that first surgery took place. He is better than before. He is an inspiration to anyone who meets him, especially me. I sat by his bed and spent time in the hospitals. Not to make me feel better. It was in some little way to help him feel better. To let him know he had people that loved him, waiting for him to beat cancer. He is my best friend, I love him like a brother, and I would never bet against him."

~

Darren is an extra-special friend in many ways. When I was sick, I remember how most people visited for a half-hour at a time and then left and said their goodbyes. There was nothing wrong with that. In fact, this is usually the case today when I visit someone in the hospital. With Darren, I could tell something was different. He would come to visit and stay for really long periods of time. We would talk when one of us needed to talk and we would just sit quietly when I did not feel up to talking.

I always wondered why he stayed so long when he had so much else he could be doing. But it sure did make me feel great that my friend never left my bedside when I needed him most. I think that after all we had been through growing up, seeing me lay in that bed fighting for my life had a profound effect on Darren.

I remember being very surprised by something that happened shortly after Darren moved in a couple houses down from ours. He was diagnosed with diabetes. He knew very little about it and I knew even less. Not too long after his diagnosis, Darren and I were getting ready to attend a basketball camp at the University of Wisconsin-Green Bay.

I remember we had a very regimented schedule between gym sessions and meals. I was nervous as a youngster who not only did not want to disappoint my coaches by being late for a session, but I also did not want to leave Darren alone, because he had to give himself an insulin shot during our lunch break. I remember having a very short time to eat and get back to the gym.

Darren was new to diabetes, and giving himself a shot in the stomach could not have been easy for a young kid. Regardless of the stringent schedule we were following, I knew staying with Darren until he was done administering his shot was the right thing to do. Regardless of the consequences that we may have faced from the UWGB coaching staff, I was not leaving my friend's side. Looking back, that is probably why he spent so much extra time by my side when I needed him most. That's what best friends do.

In the February 16, 2004, issue of *ESPN The Magazine*, I ran across an Adidas advertisement I used to read when I could tell my attitude was declining. It read: "Impossible is just a big word thrown around by small men who find it easier to live in the world they have been given rather than to explore the power they have to change it. Impossible is not a fact. It's an opinion. Impossible is not a declaration. It's a dare. Impossible is potential. Impossible is temporary. Impossible is nothing." This quote was from Muhammad Ali.

My thought at that time was beating cancer was not impossible. While it was never easy, I believe my attitude was a difference maker in my battle against cancer. Another quote I really like is from Walt Emerson. He said, "What lies behind us and what lies before us are tiny matters compared to what lies within us." This quote always reminds me to either give up or get up.

Big people overcome big obstacles. Throughout my journey with cancer, I was able to meet a lot of "big" people. I was blessed to meet a network of amazing people who taught me how to survive.

I know for a fact the challenges cancer presented to me are the very things that have driven me to start STINGCANCER and make a difference in the world. They say adversity paves the way for success, and my struggle with cancer is the chip on my shoulder. The battle against cancer is no doubt intimidating.

The network of friends and fellow survivors I was able to build were no doubt key to my survival. The people that were facing cancer just like I was were some of the strongest and most amazing people I have ever met.

Chapter 6

The Effects of Brain Cancer

At one point during my hospital stay in Chicago, I remember overhearing someone say, "Any of these three things could kill him." At the time, I was not sure what "three things" they were talking about, but I now am pretty sure they were referring to the brain cancer, the stroke and the meningitis.

A stroke is a loss of brain function due to a disturbance in the blood supply to the brain, especially when it occurs quickly. A stroke affects physical, cognitive and emotional functioning. Meningitis is an inflammation of the protective membranes covering the brain and spinal cord, collectively known as the meninges.

Both of these issues were likely contributors to the many challenges I faced as a cancer survivor. I had memory deficits that included, and still do include, a great loss of my short-term memory. I had many vision issues that are also still a challenge today.

I was left a beaten and battered man after my hospital stay. Aside from a lazy eye, numerous scars on my head and a noticeable limp, what was going on inside of me was much worse.

The "what if" question pretty much summarizes my experience with brain cancer and all its effects. Throughout my cancer journey, the "what if" questions ranged from bitterness to doubt to ultimately a tool in building confidence. While that may sound weird, the "what if" question defined my journey with cancer from the beginning to the end, with all the major ups and downs throughout.

Low mood, or even depression, is one of the most common side effects of cancer survival. Research has indicated that between 25 percent and 40 percent of people may go through some depression after cancer.

I have experienced this in many ways, dating back to the day I was diagnosed with cancer. Anger and frustration often come to the forefront when I am unable to remember something I think I should be able to. What if I never had brain cancer? Why was I the one picked for this horrendous experience? Why has my life been turned upside down?

Sometimes cancer survivors feel this way almost as soon as treatment ends, while it might hit others months or even years later. What if cancer would have never entered into my brain? Wouldn't my life be so much easier? There are many reasons why your mood might plummet after treatment, but the basic summary is simple.

You have been through a very tough experience, physically and emotionally, and it takes time to recover. Cancer survivors are often left depressed, exhausted and angry. I was extremely angry that cancer stripped me of so many things, especially the two years it took me to fully re-enter society. And how about all the doubts I still carry with me today?

Cancer survivors need to know they are not mentally ill, they are not ungrateful or weak and they do not automatically require professional help – though they may find this useful.

It is okay if they are just feeling sad. Our own expectations as survivors about life after cancer also play a part. Often, people who are going through cancer treatment make deals with themselves about what they'll do if and when they get the all-clear. I remember doing this all the time. What if I get a clean bill of health some day? What if I hear those words, "You are cancer free"?

But the pressure to make the most of life can, and often does, backfire. It can feel overwhelming. And this can leave one very confused, lost and low. Needless to say, your body also has taken a huge hit.

You may be scarred and shaken up. You may have suffered enormously. You may feel overwhelmed by side effects such as fatigue, mobility difficulties, pain and discomfort. On top of this, your general strength and fitness will probably have diminished. The Victorians had a concept called convalescence. They recognized that after a major illness, it takes someone time to recover and regain their strength.

But over the years – maybe because of the amazing advances in medical treatments – we've somehow lost this valuable idea. The expectation these days is you should be raring to go the moment you are discharged (or as soon as the time between follow-up appointments is lengthened).

Instead of telling yourself you shouldn't feel low, allow yourself time to feel this way. Sadly, you can't pack yourself off to a Victorian clinic in the Swiss Alps, but try to work out how to look after yourself while you convalesce.

Many cancer survivors are a very mixed bag of emotions. Rather than being relieved, many feel angry about why they had to suffer and the treatment they had to endure. Yes, I survived and I'm immensely relieved about that. But to suggest I'm lucky to have to have gone through four brain surgeries, chemotherapy, radiation, and years of therapy and brain retraining is a little hard to swallow at times. What if cancer did not knock me off my feet for the better part of two years? How much farther along would I be in life?

Also, I believe all cancer survivors still feel threatened. Although cancer is no longer an immediate danger, it might still feel close by. When you reach the end of your active treatment phase, even though it's obviously what you have been longing for, you can end up feeling lost, even helpless. The scariest thought is, "What if it comes back?"

When active treatment ends, people often begin to look backward, trying to work out what caused their cancer. It's common to go over and over this. If you smoked, drank too much alcohol or did any of the numerous carcinogenic things that people do every day, then you might feel regret and guilt. I still ask myself: "What if I didn't drink so much soda?" "What if I didn't shovel coal in that power plant the summer after high school?" "What if I would have exercised more?" "What if I did something to cause my brain cancer?"

You may also feel angry at yourself. Furthermore, other people's expectations can be frustrating. Whether they assume you'll instantly spring back into your normal life or insist on treating you like a fragile flower, it's common to feel misunderstood. What if they were in my shoes for a day? Maybe then they would understand.

Anger is not always bad. There are certain situations where it's useful to get angry. It can help you respond quickly to a threat or motivate you to challenge something unfair or make sure your needs are met. The moment anger met that chip on my shoulder is when I began building the tenacity to survive.

However uncontrolled, over-the-top or misplaced anger is difficult not just for you, but for the people around you. Battling the disease physically and emotionally can leave many people exhausted. Fatigue isn't like any tiredness you've had in the past. It affects you both physically and mentally. It can be overwhelming. I remember feeling guilty, asking myself, "What if I should be doing more to battle this cancer?"

Fatigue is also the most common – not to mention the most frequently ignored – side effect of cancer and its treatment. Fatigue is a physical and mental response to the stresses and treatments that cancer brings. It is also a known side effect of certain medications used in chemotherapy and radiation.

It can take a surprisingly long time to get over these. Other causes include ongoing medication and changes in your immune system or hormone levels. Your body is also likely to be out of condition. This can make you feel drained and lacking in energy, as can disrupted sleep, which is very common among cancer survivors. Your body has taken a huge hit and needs to build itself back up.

Living with cancer is an experience that can affect every part of your life. In addition to the effect cancer has on my body, it has also affected my mind and spirit. I had a lot of emotional reactions to all of these changes.

When my cancer treatment ended, the emotional effects continued and a lot of new problems surfaced. The roller coaster of emotions during my battle against cancer lingered on for years after. In my case, it is almost eighteen years as of this writing, and the brain game I still play with cancer is an ongoing, everyday thing. There is no one type of emotional response to cancer survivorship. Each survivor is different and so is each experience.

You will most likely experience a mix of emotional reactions, and some may be positive. For example, you might feel satisfaction about personal relationships that have deepened or discover increased confidence that comes with finding strengths within yourself.

On the other hand, some emotional reactions might be uncomfortable or confusing. At times, you may feel overwhelmed by conflicting feelings. You are not alone if this is how you feel during your cancer journey. For me, managing my emotions was as difficult as dealing with the medical issues.

I agree that the emotional battle against cancer oftentimes equals the physical battle. It is a common experience to have changes in emotions or moods throughout the experience with cancer. For example, at the time of my diagnosis, I was fearful, sad and worried. After deciding on a treatment plan, I felt more confident.

During treatment, I had many changes in my mood. Cancer survivors often describe this time as an emotional roller coaster – some days you may feel "up" and other days feel "down." I can honestly say I have lived on this roller coaster for the last eighteen years since my diagnosis.

After cancer treatment ends, many survivors are surprised to find they continue to experience changes in their emotions or mood. For some, completing active treatment may bring a time of emotional distress. Some survivors describe the time after treatment as one of the most emotional – and unusual – periods of their lives.

There may also be similar reactions adjusting to life after treatment. Understanding these emotions can help you manage them and feel more confident about survivorship. During treatment and recovery, I felt I was always protected by someone: my family, friends, doctors, nurses and other support staff. When it was over, and real life was waiting for me to jump back in, I found that to be a very difficult transition. What if I was not ready?

You may have all, none or only a few of these feelings and reactions. Every survivor feels and responds differently. Knowing these types of emotional reactions are common may be helpful to you. This can be a starting point for living well and accepting all types of feelings.

Many survivors expect to be thrilled and feel relieved after cancer treatment ends – and some do feel this way. I, however, was surprised to find there can be uncomfortable feelings and unanswered questions such as: What if the cancer is not gone for good? What if I have other health problems from the cancer or the treatment? Shouldn't I feel completely happy now that the treatment is done? What is going to happen now? What should I do now that I no longer see my cancer care team on a regular basis?

Emotions often surface unexpectedly. Knowing what some of these emotions are can help you understand what you are experiencing and help you find ways to manage your reactions. Until now, you may have placed your energy into managing the crisis of the diagnosis and treatment. Your focus was likely on finding a health care team, choosing the best treatment options and getting through the treatments. You may have put off paying attention to your feelings about the cancer experience.

You may have read and heard a lot about the physical and practical aspects of cancer and what you might expect to happen. However, you might not have read or heard as much about any emotional stress you could experience. Emotional effects are frequently overlooked in discussions about important side effects of treatment and survivorship.

Family members, friends and even your health care team may be ready to celebrate the victory of your beating cancer. They may expect you to get back to normal and get on with your life. Acknowledging fears or sadness when others are celebrating your success can be difficult.

When cancer treatment ends, you might feel excited about your future. You are likely to feel relieved treatment is over and ready to move on with your life. On the other hand, you could feel worried about the future, angry that you had cancer, or embarrassed that you had to rely on others for help and support. Many people have mixed feelings.

I had and still have very mixed feelings. Will the cancer come back? Fear of recurrence is one of the most common concerns for me. You might feel especially worried about the cancer coming back if you continue to have symptoms or if you have long-term effects from the treatment.

You may also feel at risk because you are no longer actively taking treatments. This may make you feel helpless against a possible recurrence of cancer. Some survivors worry their medical condition is not being watched as closely by the health care team during follow-up appointments as it was during active treatment.

I used to foolishly wish they could give me just a little bit more radiation or chemotherapy just to be sure. Some survivors say the time right after treatment ends is filled with insecurity and anxiety. You may worry something bad is about to happen.

Perhaps it feels like the threat of cancer coming back is constantly hanging over your head. Certain occurrences may cause you to feel anxious, such as health care follow-up appointments. The symptoms of common illnesses, like the flu or a cold, might be stressful.

You may find questions about how the cancer experience will affect your future cause you to feel anxious. Talk with loved ones and members of your health care team about your concerns. Ask for a referral to a licensed social worker or counselor to help you find ways deal with worries.

If you experienced physical changes during cancer treatment, you may worry about how you look to other people. Many survivors feel differently about body image after cancer and treatment. Your sense of who you are and how others see you can be challenged as you adjust to post-treatment survivorship. This was a huge hurdle for me, as I found myself bald, 65 pounds lighter, and blemished with a scarred head and a lazy eye.

Sadness is a feeling of unhappiness, unrest or mental suffering. These types of emotions can be caused by an unexpected change, stressful situations or a loss of some kind. Some find sadness to be one of the most surprising of all the post-treatment emotional effects. There may be expectations about feeling happy about surviving cancer treatment. But for me, sadness was a factor. Why me? What if this never happened to me?

Feeling sad is a common response, especially in the early months after treatment ends. During the period when you had to focus your energy on the cancer diagnosis or treatment, you may not have had a chance to let down and really think about the changes that were happening in your life. There may have been losses that were painful and hard to accept, and feeling sad is a normal response during a time of adjustment. All the physical and emotional changes in my life caused me to have many moments of sadness.

After cancer is diagnosed, it is natural to feel unsure about different aspects of life. For example, the condition of your health can be a primary area of concern. You may find yourself becoming nervous as your follow-up appointments or important anniversary dates get closer, such as the date of diagnosis or the date you completed treatment.

Cancer survivors sometimes worry more than usual about health concerns. Having a cold or headache may raise concerns. It may feel challenging to try to make plans for the future. Even though uncertainty affects people in different ways, all cancer survivors live with some uncertainty about their future.

At times, cancer can leave you feeling cheated out of the chance to have a normal life. Physical or emotional after-effects of treatment may lead to anger when reminded of losses that occurred because of cancer. I was very angry that my inability to focus, concentrate and remember important things were effects of my cancer.

While doctors and counselors are great resources, I found using your unique support group of friends and family usually help us the most when it comes to dealing with the effects of cancer. After all, these are the people who know us best. I was able to get close to and confide in those who were closest to me. While I benefitted from all my doctors, nurses and therapists, it ultimately was my own personal team of friends and family that helped me beat cancer.

Chapter 7

Surviving Cancer

It is said by many that life is a game. If this is true, then no doubt cancer is the Super Bowl. In most areas of life, we are given the lesson and then we take the test. In grade school, we typically spend a week learning about an idea or topic, and then at the end of the week we are tested on the subject.

In college, we go through a semester learning different lessons along with strategies to retain that knowledge. At the end of each particular unit, we usually are assessed through a final exam. In life, typically we are educated through different lessons and then we take the test. A professional golfer does not go into the Masters each year without practicing and learning all the environmental aspects of the course he will play.

An NFL quarterback does not go into a football game without taking an entire week scouting the opponent, taking care of his body to prevent injuries, and attending all team meetings and practices leading up to that week's big challenge. In life, preparation also is the key element.

Cancer is not life. Cancer is different. When you hear those three words, "You have cancer," you realize what you thought life is has just been turned over and is lying flat on its back. You are in the game of your life and no one has given you a scouting report. Whether you like it or not, you are at the starting line to the rest of your life. We, as people with cancer, have to decide whether we are victims or survivors.

As Dr. Seuss's famous quote goes, "You have brains in your head. You have feet in your shoes. You can steer yourself in any direction you choose." This words ring so true to cancer survivors. While you are ultimately the person who decides if you are going to do everything you can to live, there are two key things I do not think any cancer survivor can do without.

The first is an amazing foundation of family and friends. The second is an attitude that will never allow you to stop surviving. Your support foundation and attitude are the two things that will help you learn the important lessons you did not get before you took the biggest test of all: cancer. Cancer is different than most everything in life.

Typically, we learn a lesson to help us face a test. With cancer it is different. We take the most crucial test of our life and if we are lucky enough to be blessed with a great group of family and friends and strong enough to keep a positive attitude, then we will learn lessons about life and ourselves that are the most invaluable and cannot be found anywhere else.

Here are the five invaluable lessons that cancer will teach you:

1) How precious and fragile life truly is

As a cancer survivor, you will learn to celebrate life every chance you get. We value the sun rising, the sun setting and everything in between. We value each day and reflect on everything we do in a whole new, enlightened manner. We realize nothing in life – and I mean nothing – can be taken for granted. The bottom line is life is the most precious gift, and cancer survivors appreciate it like they never had before.

2) **How our attitude will determine more than anything else in life**

I believe life is 10 percent what happens to us and 90 percent how we react to what happens to us. Our attitude is the habit of the way we think. It affects how we feel and in turn how we act, and most importantly, how we face challenges. It is important to know you can't always choose what happens *to* you, but you can choose what happens *in* you. I read once that the happiest people in life don't have the best of everything, but they try to make the best of everything. Cancer survivors know the challenge of cancer is simply a temporary test of our resolve and ability.

3) **How no one is invincible or immune to cancer**

One of the most valuable lessons for me was cancer does not discriminate. I never thought I would get cancer. I was a young, vibrant college student who played football and was on the dean's list. Lance Armstrong, Deanna Favre and many more seemingly indestructible people are diagnosed with cancer every day. Cancer can invade anyone's body, but it can't take your spirit.

4) **How your friends and family are so important to your journey to survival**

I know for a fact I would not have made it through my experience without the deep love and compassion from all my friends and family members. While it is true some people who you believe to be very close to you may shy away during your fight, you will ultimately become closer to those friends and family members who don't flinch the day you tell them you have cancer. More importantly, they don't leave your side throughout your entire journey with cancer. Thank you to all those people who have been with me since the day of my diagnosis and are still here by my side today. You are truly the most special people I know.

5) How you now see "The Big Picture"

The key to enjoying life is not always striving for the prize or reward. It is realizing the true rewards in life are all the wonderful things that happen to us on a daily basis. We have to appreciate all the small victories along the way.

Here is how I think of S-U-R-V-I-V-O-R-S:

S - Strong You are strong because you had the courage to fight against an opponent that at first you may have been afraid to confront.

U - Unique You are unique because you are part of a group you did not willingly join. You will soon find you are part of a very special network of some of the most courageous people you will ever know.

R - Relentless Cancer survivors are the most relentless people I know. They have a special spirit that is unchallenged and an absolute refusal to use the words "I can't." Rightfully so, a cancer survivor believes anything is possible, because surviving cancer is our greatest and proudest achievement.

V - Vibrant Cancer survivors are the most vibrant people I have ever been around. They have the most amazing attitudes about everything, good or otherwise. I bet if you randomly selected five people and put them in front of me and told me to identify which one of them was a cancer survivor, I could tell just by the special look on their face. Cancer survivors go through their days with a special glow that encompasses their everyday smile. It is truly something that if you look really close, you see something special that is only in survivors.

I - Inspirational You as a survivor have been blessed with the gift of being able to inspire the otherwise uninspired. Typically, people facing a major challenge like cancer find it difficult to take solace in the words that come from someone who has not gone through the same trials and tribulations. However, someone who has beaten cancer has the ability to inspire other victims and turn them into survivors.

V - Victorious Enough said.

O - Outlasting You as a cancer survivor have outlasted a disease that hundreds of thousands of people are unable to beat. You will continue to overcome obstacles that come your way. Your confidence should be unwavering, as you have already faced one of life's biggest challenges and tackled it head on.

R - Responsibility As a survivor, we have a responsibility to improve the lives of others and help them become survivors.

While we typically look at a survivor as someone who remains alive despite being exposed to life-threatening danger, I have a different outlook on who true survivors are. I think a survivor is somebody with great powers of endurance; somebody who shows a great will to live or a great determination to overcome difficulties and carry on. Someone who battles the beast known as cancer.

Through my journey with cancer, I have met many people who have inspired me. These are people who refused to ever give in or give up. They battled cancer over and over again. No matter how hard they may have been knocked down, they kept getting back up.

These are the people who, despite their own struggles, always seemed to be there to help others in need first. These are people who, no matter how sick they may have been, never complained. These were people who refused to let cancer get the best of them.

Instead, they did the best they could despite cancer. These people are the reason someone like me is still here today. While they may have eventually fell victim to their own cancer, the number of other people they inspired with their journey is countless. Whether they were close friends of mine, colleagues, students in class or people I only met a handful of times, I cannot count the many fellow cancer survivors who inspired me and made me believe I could beat the beast known as cancer. Some of these survivors are still with us, but many of them are angels watching over us in heaven.

While the concept of survivors up above is difficult to grasp for some, I have no doubt some of the strongest survivors are those who may not be here on earth anymore. Because of the profound effect they had on so many people, they cannot be called anything but survivors.

Survivor Stories

Here are two stories of people I consider true survivors:

Brittany Cayemberg, strong and determined, began her battle with neuroblastoma in March 1999 at a very young age. Physicians at Mayo Clinic in Rochester, Minnesota, performed her first surgery, but the cancer recurred in March 2004. She endured another surgery at Children's Hospital of Wisconsin in Milwaukee, followed by radiation at St. Vincent Hospital in Green Bay.

During her time in radiation treatments, she befriended several elderly patients also undergoing radiation, giving them hope and inspiration – all when she was only in fourth grade. Her wish was to just be a "normal" girl in school, not the girl with cancer. Things were looking up for her until March 2007, when the cancer struck again.

Treatment options were limited, but she pushed through her time in New York and Philadelphia in an attempt to fight this disease any way she could, forgoing the pain and additional surgery.

Brittany didn't let the cancer stop her from trying to be just a "normal" girl. She made it back to school for the end of eighth grade, dressing up for the last day of school that year with her friends and taking a limousine ride as a rite of passage to high school, again hoping that she could start high school "normal," like her peers.

Treatments caused her to miss weeks of school. However, her peers were there to support her and even voted for her to be on the homecoming court ,where she was able to smile throughout the parade, football game and dance – finally feeling "normal."

Brittany's strength and determination were to be admired as she continued to maintain a 4.0 grade point average while being involved in orchestra, soccer, and the Preble STINGCANCER group as an advisor.

She devoted countless hours to supporting others who were battling cancer, all while she struggled through the pain of her own cancer. She loved life, country music, purple Gatorade, Laffy Taffy, tacos, macaroni and cheese and Fazoli's restaurant.

Brittany earned her wings February 21, 2010, after eleven years of fighting. All who knew Brittany were truly inspired by her courage and service to others while just trying to be "normal." The world was certainly better for having had Brittany in it. Normal she was not. Extraordinary she was.

~

Deanna Sundstrom was a math teacher at Preble and a STINGCANCER advisor. Her spirit and the way she battled cancer inspired so many people. She was a cancer survivor. While she battled cancer for years, she always put the needs of others battling cancer before her own. She was an amazing wife and mother. She was the most pure-of-heart person most of us have ever known.

She saw the good in everyone. Deanna gave everyone who crossed her path the benefit of the doubt. She completely lived for her family. Deanna battled leiomeiosarcoma (LMS), a very rare form of cancer. She battled this beast for years. In fact, when she finally had to stop fighting, we held a STINGCANCER meeting so she could explain to everyone what was happening. Over three hundred students showed up for that meeting.

A week later, when she was in her final days, over two hundred faculty members and students showed up at her house to say goodbye. She sat in a chair on her front lawn and gave every last person a hug, a kiss and well wishes. I remember that day like it was yesterday.

She was the person that taught so many of us how to help others, regardless of our own personal situation. And now there she was, in her last hours, and she was worried only about how everyone else was handling her impending death. It was the most courageous, selfless act I had ever seen.

On that day she gave me one of the best compliments I have ever received. When I bent over to embrace her, to tell her I loved her and was going to miss her, she said, "Nick, I love you, too – and thanks for being my husband at work." At the time, we both laughed.

However, we had a special bond, as we both were cancer survivors and we shared a fierce tenacity in fighting the effects of cancer on ourselves and others. While I lost a dear friend that week, my friendship with Deanna only fueled the passion I had for STINGCANCER.

Those two instances alone, the last meeting at school and that day at her house, showed the mighty effect she had on everyone she touched. Her spirit and her intense drive to help others set an amazing example not only for our students, but also all the adults in our school building.

Deanna is truly the epitome of a survivor in heaven. While she may be up above, the effect she had on so many other people and her willingness to put everyone before herself makes her a survivor in my book. Preble's math department named the math lab in her honor because of the teacher and person she was, Highlighting the pillars of her legacy: The Deanna Sundstrom Math Lab: Believe, Have Faith, Serve.

Working with Deanna as a fellow cancer survivor was probably the most eye-opening, inspiring experience in my life. In my cubicle at Preble hangs the last email I received from my dear friend. It reads:

> *"Hi Nick, I hope you know that from the bottom of my soul, I love you. You are the inspiration to continue the battle against cancer. God's love and strength to you, Deanna."*

I would argue the opposite. Deanna was the inspiration for all of us at Preble High School to continue the battle against cancer.

Chapter 8

My Life After Cancer

I entered St. Norbert College a muscular, 220-pound, football-playing, curly-haired, dean's list student. While the knee injury had affected me somewhat emotionally and physically, I had no idea the transformation I was facing before I stepped back on the SNC campus after being away, fighting for my life. I had lost sixty pounds, had a lazy eye from the stroke, and my head was full of scars from multiple surgeries.

I had been a student with a full academic load of sixteen credits per semester, football practice, weightlifting, film study and hours of homework each night. It was natural to burn the midnight oil, cramming for an exam until 3 a.m. and then waking up at 7 a.m., going to class at 8 a.m., acing the exam and completing the rest of my day with the same ease and success.

Now I was facing much different circumstances. My doctors had told me because of my stroke, I had lost a great deal of short-term memory, among other things. They told me I immediately had to discontinue my two most memory-intensive classes and go on a part-time, eight-credit course load. This news was very difficult to handle.

This was not my style at all, and I still had not come to grips with the way this brain tumor and its subsequent effects had derailed me and my lifestyle. I was a business communication major, and my two most memory-intensive courses were in the communications department.

When I began to realize I could study days only to remember nothing once the intimidating "blue book" essay booklet was sitting on my desk, I was devastated. My memory and ability to focus were now just more things cancer had taken from me.

So now I had to go talk to the most important business communication professors on campus. I had to tell them because of the heavy amount of content in their courses, my doctor had recommended I drop their high-level, memory-intensive classes. This meant I had the daunting task of setting up meetings with these two men and telling them because of my health situation, I needed to drop their courses and take them at a later time when my memory would hopefully be improved.

When I approached the first professor's office, I was nervous and scared. This was my first visit to campus in months and my appearance was not the only thing that had changed dramatically. My confidence and "swagger" were completely gone. No longer was I the football player, the dean's list student or one of the popular guys on campus. I was a fragile fragment of my former self who was about to attempt to reclaim my old life a little bit at a time.

He greeted me and I immediately felt at ease and comfortable. We talked for about a half an hour and he hugged me, shed a tear, and gave me his very best wishes as I departed his office. I felt like a load had been lifted and things were actually going to be okay. Maybe eventually I could make it all the way back? Maybe I was not as different as before as I thought I was.

About an hour later I had my second meeting. As I waited outside this man's office, I felt a newfound confidence, as my previous meeting had gone so well. I entered his office and again related the story of my summer, the brain tumor, the stroke, the meningitis infection in my brain stem. I told this second professor how all these things had affected my ability to focus and concentrate. More importantly, I told him how I had lost most of my short-term memory.

In my mind, I expected a similar response from the second professor as the one I had got from the first. However, the response I got blew my mind, and still does. He looked me in the eyes and said, "Well Nick, I am very sorry for what you have had to endure since I last saw you. But what you are telling me is that you are quitting my class. And Nick, I have a rule in my life: That I do not associate with quitters."

What? In three short sentences this egotistical man had trivialized my experience of fighting for my life into being a quitter? Was he out of his mind? Did he have any clue I had had four brain surgeries? Did he know I underwent eighteen weeks of grueling chemotherapy? How about another sixteen weeks of radiation? Did he know I was in the middle of four months of physical therapy, three months of occupational therapy and three months of speech therapy? How about the monthly sessions with my newly assigned neuropsychologist that I would continue to see for four years?

How could one man totally deflate my confidence in one short conversation? I do not think I have ever been so angry. The moment he looked me in the eye and called me a quitter, he lit a very strong flame inside of me.

Even though I was in the middle of finishing my interpersonal communications degree at St. Norbert, I think I knew my ultimate destiny was teaching the moment this man called me a quitter. In that moment, he exemplified exactly what a teacher should not be. All his degrees and experience made him a professor and a doctor (surely not the kind that helps people), but they did not make him a teacher. I truly have to thank him for teaching me one lesson that I will never forget, and that is how not to be a teacher.

Meanwhile, I was gaining value in my life from coaching. Coaching is where I was finding meaning. I was shaping my future and sorting out my priorities without even realizing it.

I coached at both Denmark and St. Norbert for two years. I also began substitute teaching while coaching. I subbed in classes ranging from kindergarten through high school and loved it. I was able to combine two of my passions: football and being in a leadership role.

Once one has a vision, a direction and a mission in life, it is time to work toward it with a passion. I needed to use my obstacles in life as fuel for my future. I began to be urged by many people around me to go back to school and pursue a degree in teaching. I was already substituting teaching and coaching and I loved it.

With no money, I was lucky enough to return to school through a graduate assistant coaching job at Lakeland College. I took twenty-two classes in two years at Lakeland, both graduate and undergraduate. I then did my student teaching at Denmark and was welcomed back to their football coaching staff.

Chapter 9

Making a Difference

"Do not follow where the path may lead.
Go instead where there is no path and leave a trail."
- Harold R. McAlindon

Why do people teach? Reasons to become a teacher are as diverse as the subjects they plan to teach. Motives range from inspiration drawn from a favorite teacher, to a sense of commitment to a community or nation, to an intellectual fascination with a given discipline, such as English literature or the physical sciences. But the most compelling reason to become a teacher is the desire to work with children. I would say it is a calling, a yearning to help children learn, watch them grow and make a meaningful difference in the world.

No doubt, the choice to become a teacher is a decision to make a significant impact on the future. The truth is, however, the profession is tremendously demanding, especially today. As new graduates become teachers, they are called upon to motivate dozens, in some cases, hundreds of students every day, teach an ever-expanding curriculum with little prep time, maintain order and promote a structured learning environment, keep up to date with a litany of administrative tasks, and spend evenings and weekends grading papers and planning lessons – not to mention stay current with educational reforms and changes in the profession.

I came from Denmark, Wisconsin, and attended Denmark High School, a school of approximately 420 students in grades 9-12. I was a football player, a basketball player, a baseball player and a golfer. Later, I was a substitute teacher there for a year and a student teacher for six months. Never did I think Denmark was a small place until I got to Green Bay Preble High School.

I earned a degree from nearby St. Norbert College in Interpersonal Communications, but after cancer, it all seemed so trivial. I needed to make a difference. My coaching experience convinced me I needed to go back to school to become a teacher.

I quit my job with the American Cancer Society and went to Lakeland College as a graduate assistant. While I was passionate about the American Cancer Society's mission, I wanted to further develop my career and uphold the fight against cancer in a stronger way. Nothing against the ACS, but deep inside of me, I knew there was a better way to make a difference.

At Lakeland, I coached football and recruited high school players to come play at the college in return for free tuition. To this day, it was the best decision I ever made. I was able to get my teaching certificate in two years. My experience as a football coach and graduate student at Lakeland was great.

Our football team included about 40 percent young men from inner-city Detroit and another 40 percent from the Upper Peninsula of Michigan, otherwise known as "Yoopers" because of the U.P. abbreviation for the region. The remaining 20 percent were local guys and a few from the

Milwaukee or Green Bay areas. I never thought a team made up of Yoopers and inner-city kids could gel so perfectly and make my experience as a football coach so satisfying. Regardless of their backgrounds, they respected and loved one another in a special way.

After a lengthy interview with eight principals from the Green Bay Area Public School District following my graduation from Lakeland, Preble principal Dr. Christopher Wagner asked me to join his staff. So the next fall, I prepared for the first major challenge since cancer, and that was becoming a teacher at Preble High School. I was hired as a special education teacher, meaning I would be spending my days with cognitively disabled students. These students had disabilities including Down syndrome, autism, cerebral palsy and many other handicaps that made their lives very challenging.

The enrollment at Denmark High School was 420 students. I was now at Preble, enrollment 2,350 students. Yes, almost six times larger. I looked at myself and said, "Toto, we're not in Kansas anymore." And if that wasn't the truth, I don't know what was.

Still suffering from the effects of my stroke, my spatial orientation was nowhere near where it should have been. No good at all. Even after spending two years with a neuropsychologist for what they had called brain-retraining sessions, my spatial orientation still remained terrible. Neither Dr. Hitch, my neuropsychologist, nor I could figure it out.

Countless times walking out of classrooms at Preble, I remember inadvertently turning the wrong way and faking it, pretending like I knew where I was going. I would walk down a hallway maybe a hundred yards out of my way, just to make sure I looked like I knew what I was doing. "Definitely not in Denmark anymore," I would say to myself every once in a while. Could I do this? Could I actually instruct and get the respect of students when I could barely figure out how to get around this massive building?

After all, the Preble building was 424,195 square feet. There were over 140 classrooms on two floors. The current ethnic breakdown of Preble includes 27 American Indian students, 104 African American students, 1,350 Caucasian students, 521 Hispanic students and 139 Southeast Asian students. The building itself was overwhelming for me in many ways, both good and bad.

The academic and extracurricular offerings at Preble rival any in the state. Academically, Preble students consistently score above the national and state averages. *U.S. News & World Report* ranked Preble as the No. 17 high school in Wisconsin. Students also have outstanding records in the areas of art, music, forensics, technology and athletics. Innovative programs include DNA testing, computer-assisted design, subject integrations and math analysis. The educational focus is to prepare students for the global environment of the next century. Preble operates a traditional eight-period schedule.

Our special education department consists of three main categories: students are cognitively disabled (CD), learning disabled (LD) or emotionally disturbed (ED). My teaching position was primarily working with the CD students. Needless to say, I could identify with these kids very easily because of what I had and was going through. These children appreciate life so much, and there are so many lessons they can teach us.

At Denmark, we had had three special-education teachers and about fifteen or sixteen special-education students. At Preble, we had a staff of special-education teachers nearly thirty strong, with over three hundred special-education students. How was I going to be able do this when I could hardly get around the building without getting lost? What about all the other effects of the stroke I have had? The memory issues? The spatial issues? Organization? How was I going to make it at Preble High School? The what-if-I-can't-do-this question turned quickly into what-if-I-can, due to the great people that made up our school building.

Wow, the effects of my brain tumor and stroke were right there at the forefront of my life. And yet I was still finding success as a teacher and a coach. What if I really could beat this beast known as cancer?

At first glance, I always thought of myself as a fairly decent-looking guy. When you get a little closer, though, you see the scars. You see the baldness. You see the effects of what had been a lengthy battle. I soon realized I was going to have to make a decision. I was either going to have to hide what happened to me or embrace it. And I was not going to hide it. Cancer had controlled me for too long, and it was time I regained control and took my life back.

Yes, I looked different. But you know what? Preble was now my home, whether I liked it or not. I was going to make it my home. I was engaged to be married, and rings aren't free. I needed to have a steady income, and I had met a beautiful girl named Maureen, whom I wanted to marry more than anything ever in my life.

So here we go! I soon learned Preble was a special place with special people. I put all those other thoughts behind me. People were embracing and involving, and they truly cared. People in leadership roles were passionate about what they did. They were passionate about teaching children and helping children grow into young adults – adults that would be successful.

I soon knew this was the place I wanted to be. It was a special place with special people. People were surprisingly open, engaging and friendly, right off the bat. I think a lot of people looked at me and wondered, "What happened to him?" The multiple scars on my head and the lazy eye were all things others wondered about. I respect Preble and its staff so much for the care they showed by saying, "Hey, if you don't mind me asking, Nick, what happened?"

This is not something that happened every day, although it began to happen a lot as I became more involved at Preble and comfortable in my situation. People got to know me and they wanted to know what happened. I realized that while it was therapeutic for me to talk about what had happened, it seemed like it was therapeutic for others to relay their stories about how they had been affected by cancer. One interaction in particular seemed to affect me more than all the others.

A member of the Preble faculty came to me and asked about the scars on my head shortly after school started. When I told her my story about my brain cancer and all I had been through, she was so incredibly thankful. She went on to tell me her neighbor's son was going through something similar with a brain tumor. She said just knowing someone survived a similar situation was going to provide her neighbor with so much hope for her son. My colleague told me she could hardly wait to get home to tell my story to her neighbor.

I noticed this mutual, therapeutic kind of endearing conversation would occur almost daily with someone new. It was really neat! Although I was a special education teacher and football coach, I began meeting people from all realms of the school: guidance counselors, custodians, monitors, paraprofessionals, even regular education students that I didn't have in my classroom.

Preble administration had done a great job making sure everybody in this very large building filled with over 2,600 people knew and appreciated each other. I think my proudest moment at Preble was when I finally realized my title there was football coach, assistant football coach, and special education teacher. But my title for life, what I was most proud of, was being a cancer survivor; proudly telling my story and listening intently to the stories of others.

Really for the first time, I had the realization that was my proudest achievement was being a cancer survivor. And it was the many people at Preble High School, just through talking to me at the water cooler or sitting down and having lunch conversations, that made me realize how proud and how lucky I am to be a cancer survivor. I often said I thought having cancer was the best thing that ever happened to me, and now I began to truly believe it because the Preble community had made such a difference in my young life.

I think inherently, every teacher wants to make a difference in their school and in the community, wherever it may be. Is that possible? That was the question I had at hand. I wanted to make a difference at school and in the Preble building. I wanted to do something that would make a difference. I also wanted to do something in the community.

After all, this was near the community where I grew up. Denmark was only about fifteen miles from where Preble High School is located on the east side of Green Bay. I wanted to do something beneficial, something that would make a difference at Preble and in the surrounding community. While I knew I made a difference in the classroom and on the football field with the kids I coached, I wanted more. I was always thinking about how I could get more involved.

I knew cancer had happened to me for a reason. I began realizing that almost everyone affected wanted to share their story in one way or another. People wanted to hear my story and they wanted to share theirs. Could there be such a thing as a group of people who share their feelings about cancer, get to know each other and make a difference in the community? How could I combine everything to make a difference in the school and the community? That was the big question.

How will administration take this? What will they think? People obviously care about my story. They want to share their stories. But this is unprecedented! No other high school in the United States had a cancer-driven awareness group. Nobody. I can't believe it! I've looked online, I've looked in books and I've made phone calls. No other high school in the nation had a cancer awareness group. Amazing!

But so many people in this building are yearning to tell their stories, to provide hope for others and gain hope from hearing the stories of others. But no other school had a cancer-driven awareness group like I was beginning to envision.

So what? We will be the first. And since our school's nickname is the Hornets – this came to me like an epiphany as I was walking down to Dr. Wagner's office to meet him about this – we are going to call ourselves STINGCANCER. And our goal will be to STINGCANCER in any way we can.

First, and foremost, we will bring together a group of students and staff members who share a common bond. Unfortunately, they most likely have been affected by cancer at some point in their lives. The STINGCANCER group will allow the Preble community an opportunity to collectively share their experiences with this horrific disease.

It can help form new friendships, but more importantly for many, it can be a form of grief support. It can become a source of comfort and solace for students and staff.

Also – and equally important – it will provide us all with an opportunity to reach out to others who are experiencing the devastating effects of cancer. The STINGCANCER group will brainstorm ideas and activities that will allow us to raise money as well as awareness for the many people suffering from cancer.

I believed the group would bring awareness and sensitivity to a subject people often don't pay attention to unless they are directly affected by it. It will involve many different types of kids. We will help out families in need and show the importance of compassion. It will bring about a sense of community, and help students and adults to see the bigger picture in life.

Using our group's funds, we will be able to make a difference for families in need. Those who suffer from cancer in our community will know they are not alone. Cancer affects all of us. Students who participate in the STINGCANCER group at Preble will see how they can help make the world a better place, simply from the acts of kindness they do for others affected by cancer. More importantly, it will show them how we are all connected.

Everyone will be able to identify with this group. Everyone knows someone who is affected by cancer in some way, shape or form. It is one of the only student groups that will hopefully have all students from all backgrounds. It will be a blend of students, who despite different interests, come together for one common cause. My hope was that students will emerge as leaders because of involvement with STINGCANCER. This is a group that staff and students will be able to work together side-by-side for a good cause.

So many of high school extra-curricular activities are only self-rewarding. This is a club where people make a difference and students can volunteer sincerely, without earning service-learning hours. Today we have so many kids volunteering only because they have to and not because they care. But in STINGCANCER, our students and staff will have a purpose together.

That all sounds great, right? Being a trail-blazer and trying to successfully implement the first-ever, high school-driven cancer awareness group was not a slam-dunk, as I may have assumed. While everyone has been affected by cancer, not everyone has experienced its vengeance like I had. Aside from that, many people who had been hit hard by cancer did not want to talk about their experiences or did not care to be as open as I was. This is understandable. Not everyone deals with the idea of cancer in the same way. For some, their experiences with cancer are something they want to keep quiet.

Maybe this is why even my principal had many reservations about me starting STINGCANCER. He was justified, pointing out that so many teachers are eager to start social groups on campus. He went on to say that many times these groups fall by the wayside and disappear after a few months. He said that was why he had initial reservations about my idea to start STINGCANCER. He said when a group gets started and then quickly falls apart, it is never a good thing for Preble. It makes Preble look bad, it makes him look bad and ultimately it makes the group's leader look bad as well.

Although he was a bit hesitant at first, Dr. Wagner gave me his blessing and support to start STINGCANCER. While that was the first step to getting this group off of the ground, there were going to be a few more hurdles ahead.

Our first meeting was scheduled and I could not have been more excited and more nervous at the same time. That day in the library, it was fourteen students and me.

I was feeling good until we met again two weeks later. In that second meeting, it was me and only nine students. What had happened to those other five? Was my wonderful idea of starting a cancer awareness group in a high school over before it started? Because of my meeting with Dr. Wagner, I was now a bit stressed out when I thought about the state of STINGCANCER after two meetings.

However, we soon found strategies to market the brand STINGCANCER throughout our school. Word began to spread from our dozen or so members. We decided to get our school more involved by having a t-shirt sale. A few months later, we held a baseball cap sale.

With the money we raised from the two fundraisers, we were able to start helping people battling cancer in the Preble community. We were able to start developing our Helping Hands branch of STINGCANCER. This facet of STIGCANCER focuses on helping people who are connected to our Preble community.

When people within our building are connected to someone battling cancer, they can fill out a "Helping Hands" form. Our group takes these forms and customizes a gift basket for the family of the person battling cancer.

We really take pride in including items in these baskets that truly are unique to each family's needs. Through Helping Hands, we are able to include gas cards, gift cards and grocery cards for places that are favorites of each specific family. These baskets also include STINGCANCER t-shirts, STINGCANCER blankets, wristbands and other items that will hopefully make each person's journey a bit smoother.

We also help hundreds of people each year by delivering "Backpacks for the Battle" to each oncology unit in Green Bay during every major holiday throughout the calendar year. These backpacks are not customized to each individual because of the sheer number that are disseminated each year. However, they are filled with all kinds of items that will help people who are going through chemotherapy or radiation.

While we receive hundreds of thank-you cards from people who are very touched by these gifts, we recently received a very unique thank you. It was not from a cancer patient. It was from a nurse who worked in one of the local oncology units in Green Bay.

She said her job is to guide patients back to the lobbies or their hospital rooms after their exhaustive treatments. She thanked us for giving her renewed energy and a passion for her job again. She said she had become so used to seeing people at their worst moments after their hellish treatments.

Being the person that presented these backpacks to the patients had made her job so much more fulfilling. She could not express in words how amazing it was to see these people's faces change when they were handed these backpacks. Her job and her life improved because she saw more smiles in a place where they had been few and far between.

STINGCANCER volunteers also help those with cancer by raking leaves, shoveling snow or planting flowers for those who are busy dealing with treatment and unable to do physical activity. All in all, we try to help in any way we can with anything someone with cancer may need.

Also, through students and their family members and friends sporting STINGCANCER gear, we are really spreading awareness of what the group is all about. The awareness was spreading through our building as well as through the Green Bay community. While what STINGCANCER was doing was new to most everyone, it was also something very needed by many people we came across.

One person in particular was Todd Darrow. He was a man in his early seventies who had no fears in life. He kept in great physical shape through his older years and very seldom had any health problems. Needless to say, Todd was shocked when he found out about his cancer and his grim chances of living much longer.

As Todd heard those three harsh words, "You have cancer," he went through all the emotions that go along with them. But Todd decided he was going to make the most of the time he had left. He found out about STINGCANCER when he received a comfort bag from us while undergoing treatment at a local oncology unit.

What started out with a thank you letter from Todd turned into a love affair between a man in his seventies and close to a hundred Green Bay Preble STINGCANCER students. Todd had hinted he would like to meet the amazing kids who were part of our group. Our group members urged our adult advisors to ask if Todd would come in and speak to them about his experiences. I am very sure none of us expected what happened next.

Todd arrived at Preble for one of our Thursday meetings dressed in a STINGCANCER shirt and hat. While our building is often viewed as intimidating to parents and other outside community members because of its size and the amount of students, Todd walked in without hesitation and bared his soul in front of our STINGCANCER group. Todd laughed and he cried.

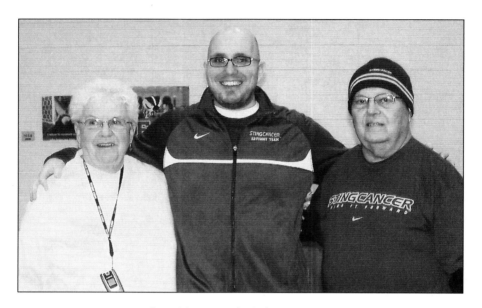

Me with Todd Darrow (right) and his wife, Rosie.

He talked about his wife, the love of his life. He spoke about living. He spoke about dying. He very quickly became part of the STINGCANCER group.

When Todd learned there were now other STINGCANCER chapters throughout the Green Bay area, he began visiting them and sharing his life lessons as well. Over time, Todd talked about everything from writing his own obituary and helping his wife pick out his coffin to trying to finish his bucket list before he was called to heaven.

Trying to fulfill his bucket list was one speech that really resonated with our group. What if we could somehow help Todd scratch all the items off that list?

Todd was a graduate of the University of Notre Dame. The most amazing and seemingly most unlikely item to get crossed off his bucket list was a trip back to Notre Dame with his brother, who was also a graduate of this famous university. Todd specifically wanted to go back to campus and pray at The Grotto of Our Lady of Lourdes. The Grotto of Our Lady of Lourdes is one-seventh the size of the famed French shrine where the Virgin Mary appeared to Saint Bernadette on eighteen occasions in 1858.

Visiting the site on one of his many trips to his native country, Notre Dame founder, Father Edward Sorin, vowed to reproduce it on the campus of his new university. A gift from Rev. Thomas Carroll, a former theology student, made it possible in 1896. Boulders from surrounding farms, most weighing two tons or more, were used in its construction.

A small piece of stone from the original grotto in France is located on the right-hand side of the shrine directly below the statue of Mary. To Notre Dame students and alumni, the Grotto is a special place to spend a few quiet moments. Especially during football weekends and finals, you might have difficulty finding a candle to light. Hundreds of students have proposed marriage here, outdoor Masses are celebrated regularly and the Rosary is prayed every day at 6:45 p.m., rain or shine.

This was an area on campus Todd cherished when he was a student. While Todd knew this item was not likely to be crossed off his list, he was the type of confident man that was always going to reach for the stars.

That is same attitude our STINGCANCER group had when we decided we were going to send Todd and his brother back to Notre Dame and his beloved Grotto. We found an amazing community member who had long supported STINGCANCER to donate his frequent flier miles for Todd's airline tickets. From there, we took care of all the other arrangements. Todd and his brother had the time of their lives, and ultimately Todd completed his bucket list with a little help from a group of special people from Preble High school known as STINGCANCER.

While Todd's story is a special one, we have helped a number of people in smaller but very significant ways. Over the last ten years we have helped over one thousand individuals who are battling cancer. And that is just the group at Preble High School. Our original intent was simply to have a small cancer awareness group at Preble that met a few times per month. However, we have branched outside of Preble through our Sting It Forward program. As of this writing, we now have STINGCANCER groups in more than twenty other schools in Northeast Wisconsin.

When our group began gaining in popularity and expanding in membership, Dr. Wagner began to caution me. He wanted to make sure I could handle the larger numbers of people that were making up the group. At one point, he called me down to his office and told me he had heard we were helping people on the west side of Green Bay. This concerned him.

Little did he know we were actually helping people as far away as Trinidad in the Caribbean and Somerset, England. One of our adult advisors, Deanna Sundstrom, had been on a service trip to Trinidad. Through a letter that was sent to her after she returned home, she found out one of her friends she had met in Trinidad was battling breast cancer. She brought her friend's story to the attention of our group and we immediately put together a customized care package for this woman and her family, and sent it off to Trinidad.

That same school year, Becky, our librarian at Preble, told me about her friend from Somerset, England, who was in a major struggle with pancreatic cancer. His name was Eddie Maguire, and he was the author of numerous Sherlock Holmes novels including *Sherlock Holmes and the Three Poisoned Pawns* and *Sherlock Holmes & the Secret Mission*.

Again, our group of amazing young people agreed we should customize a basket for Eddie and send it off to England.

Eddie was so overwhelmed by the generosity from people he never met. He sent us numerous thank you cards with very thoughtful messages. On top of that, he asked Becky if he could have my phone number. Shortly after, Eddie and I talked for the first time and realized we had a lot in common. Not only had we both had cancer, but we both wanted to fight this beast any way we could.

Even though Eddie was a well-known author, all he wanted to talk about was cancer and how we were going to end it. He praised our STINGCANCER group and was always eager to learn more about what we were doing.

We talked about the prevalence of cancer in America and England. We talked about life. We talked about how it did not matter who you were, what your age was or how you necessarily lived your life. Cancer simply does not discriminate. While our conversations were lively and heartwarming, they did not last forever. After a few unsuccessful attempts to get ahold of Eddie, I began to become concerned. That day when Becky showed up in my classroom, I knew something was wrong. She told me she had received a call the night before and cancer had taken Eddie's life.

While Dr. Wagner was wary of how our group was evolving, he was very supportive and only looking out for our best interests. He was always very supportive of STINGCANCER. As we evolved, he recognized the need for a group like ours.

I will always be thankful for Dr. Wagner's blessing to start STINGCANCER. If he would not have had the courage to give me the green light to start STINGCANCER, my life and the lives of many other people would be much different.

I will never forget when I began getting calls from nearby schools complimenting us on the way we were improving the lives of people we helped and making a difference in the community. The question from many of them then was, "How can we start a STINGCANCER group?"

I cannot tell you how flattering that was for all of us. We were finding out the impact we had made in the community was so strong, other schools could not wait to learn how to do the same thing. It started with De Pere and Brillion, and my alma mater, Denmark, was the third school.

These groups were started by other teachers and students who wanted to make a difference. There was no mass letter sent to all schools in Wisconsin. There was not a seminar given at teachers' conferences around the state. It was simply a matter of really passionate adults, along with some really strong young leaders, who had been affected by cancer and wanted to change the world in a small way.

Our hope is there will be STINGCANCER groups throughout the United States and maybe even around the world. The combination of passionate adults and young people who want to be leaders is what is going to make our hope a reality.

The groups at other local schools all have strong student involvement as well. Today, STINGCANCER can boast about one thousand student participants at more than twenty schools. While I never intended this evolution, it really evolved because of a group of passionate people who refuse to let cancer get the best of them. Our motto is STING the Beast, and that is exactly what we intend to do.

Green Bay Preble's STINGCANCER Awareness Group is a passionate and committed collaboration of high school students, faculty and staff dedicated to reducing the effects of cancer by initiating and supporting programs and activities for the school and its surrounding community.

The STINGCANCER Creed

We believe in life.

Your life and the lives or your family and friends.

We believe in living every minute with a heartfelt passion and an intense commitment to it.

We believe in putting intense energy into your life, channeled with a fierce aggression.

We believe in focus: staying strong in mind and soul.

Knowledge is power. Commitment to the cause breeds success. Attitude strengthens our lives.

This is the "STINGCANCER Awareness Team."

We can be there whenever you need us.

Hopefully, we can lessen the tears and help the anger subside.

If we can brighten your day, then we have done our job.

We believe in providing care and compassion.

Not pity.

We know this is no time to pull any punches.

You are in the fight for your life, and we want to help.

We are about the fight against cancer.

Chapter 10

Starting Your Own STINGCANCER Group

One of the modus operandi with STINGCANCER has been to operate at 212 degrees.

This idea may be familiar to some and unfamiliar to others. The concept is that at 211 degrees, water is hot. At 212 degrees, it boils. And with boiling water comes steam. And steam can power a locomotive. The idea is that seemingly small things can make a tremendous difference.

STINGCANCER will make a difference in your life and the lives of those battling cancer. It will also be life-changing for the students who are in your group.

Becoming a STINGCANCER leader will absolutely assure life-altering, positive effects in your life. As teachers, we want our students to always take the extra step in finishing homework or making sure a new student has help getting around school during their first days.

While being an advisor or leader with an STINGCANCER group may seem like a daunting task, I can absolutely guarantee it will the best, most rewarding experience of your life.

I have often felt rewarded by steps taken, goals achieved and dreams realized by students in the classroom. However, I have never been prouder or more awestruck than by the challenges that our STINGCANCER students have met.

Exponential rewards are possible by taking that extra step. Educating students beyond the classroom is what STINGCANCER is all about, learning those life lessons that are not possible anywhere else. I have coached football for fifteen years and taught for eleven years, and I have never seen such amazing displays of teamwork, leadership and selflessness as I have by students in STINGCANCER. The group truly brings out the best in everyone.

It goes beyond textbooks and laboratory manuals to creating experiences that enable students to use their minds and their hearts in a much more hands-on manner. STINGCANCER is modernizing education by removing the walls between school and real life, and we are changing lives with the same innovation, leadership and tenacity that many not-for-profit groups have. What separates us is we do it with passionate teachers and students who want to be difference-makers in this world. When a group of passionate teachers and energized students come together for a common cause, the possibilities are truly endless.

Knowing how overwhelmed, and in many cases over-burdened, teachers are in today's schools, the easy answer is to say no. You may feel there is no way you can add the responsibility of being a leader for a STINGCANCER group at your school onto everything you are already doing.

However, STINGCANCER is different. This is the opportunity that is worth stepping out of your comfort zone. I once heard the only thing that stands between a person and what they want in life is the will to try it and the faith to believe it possible.

If you want an opportunity to guide young people and watch their passion for improving the lives of those affected by cancer grow and mature, then do not pass up the chance to lead a STINGCANCER group at your school.

If you believe the fight against cancer is worthwhile, your belief will no doubt fuel enthusiasm in your students. That enthusiasm fires our souls and lifts our spirits. When students and school staff come together in STINGCANCER, not only is your school building a better place, but the community around your school will improve as well.

Surrounding schools and businesses will be motivated to support you and feel a responsibility to help you in any way they possibly can. After all, no one is immune to the effects of cancer.

While we all feel as if we have too much going on, I have found that making time and taking the extra step to be involved in STINGCANCER is the best professional decision I ever made.

It is pretty simple, actually! It comes down to eliminating the distractions around you. When did you last evaluate the tasks you do every day against what's most important to you? When did you last evaluate them against who is most important to you?

You have goals. You have time. You have energy. Where should it be invested?

You can start a STINGCANCER group and become a STINGCANCER advisor at your school with a few short steps: First and foremost is to have that passionate person who wants to fight cancer, help their students break down barriers and teach lessons that go far beyond the classroom. That person is YOU!

Before contacting your administrator for permission, my recommendation would be to discuss your plans with a few colleagues who may want to assist you with the group or you know will be there for support if needed.

Next, I would recommend having a few solid students to whom you can disclose your plans and get feedback. Your students will not only be excited about the prospect of a school-driven cancer awareness group in their school, they will also have valuable ideas from their unique student perspective.

Make sure you customize your STINGCANCER group. We at Preble are the original group and the "STING" came from our mascot, the hornet. Currently we have more than twenty other groups at various schools in Northeast Wisconsin. While they are all STINGCANCER groups, they each customize their school's group with a sub-logo. For example, Brillion High School in Brillion, Wisconsin, is surrounded by a community that is very passionate about hunting. Hence their logo looks like this:

"Brillion STINGCANCER, *Hunting for a Cure.*" This allows them to customize their unique group but still operate under the larger umbrella of groups involved in STINGCANCER.

In order to receive support and assistance throughout the beginning of your journey with STINGCANCER, please email Nick Nesvacil at nwnesvacil@gbaps.org.

Find a home base in your school building where you and your students will begin to change lives on a weekly basis.

Brainstorm potential community involvement. Think about local businesses and parent groups that are able to help you get started. After all, once your group gets started, your surrounding community will be overwhelmed with the lives you are changing. Getting some key people from your community to understand what you are proposing will go a long way in having your idea approved by your principal. It also will help you gain further support from the outside community down the road.

If you find it a struggle to gain funds, have a fundraising activity (i.e. shirt sale, family fun day, etc.) contact me and learn about our Sting It Forward stipend program.

With your awareness of the power of STINGCANCER now comes responsibility and action. Here is your opportunity to improve the lives of your students and yourself. We all know cancer is not going away, and neither is STINGCANCER. In fact, our hope is someday soon, STINGCANCER groups will be a common sight in schools across America. It will be a natural part of the school experience like basketball, band and student council. You know have the ability to help make that happen. Are you ready to make a difference?

Picture yourself on the bulletin board of life as unique and significant. After reading the STINGCANCER mission and creed, you should feel compelled to become a STINGCANCER leader at your school. Now that you know what STINGCANCER is and what it is all about, it is time to apply it to your life. Because when you do, exciting things begin to happen.

Aside from being part of the strongest, most powerful team your school has ever seen, you are now going to be absolutely fulfilled on a daily basis by the people you will meet and the lives you are going to have the opportunity to improve.

Starting a STINGCANCER group at your school through our STING It Forward program or joining an existing STINGCANCER group will help you immediately find more joy and fulfillment in your life. You will begin to perform everything you do at a higher level, because inside your heart, you will know you are contributing to something much greater than yourself: the fight against cancer. As a byproduct of your membership with this group, you will have a new, positive feeling about yourself and your place in life.

Our Preble group has found numerous ways to fundraise, and more importantly, we have found there are endless ways to help those battling cancer and their families. We have done a lot of different things over the years to bring the community together and increase our funds at the same time. We have held dinner galas and we held carnival-like family fun days. We also raise a lot of awareness by selling dynamic STINGCANCER gear such as t-shirts and hats.

These events not only allow us to raise money to help people with cancer, they also bring our students, school and surrounding community together. Everyone has been touched by cancer in one way or another, and it is amazing when a STINGCANCER school and its surrounding community come together to fight the effects of cancer.

Many STINGCANCER groups assist at outside community events. Whether it is helping other cancer awareness groups like the American Cancer Society or providing manpower for a specific family who is planning a benefit for a loved one, our kids are willing to help in any way they can. There are endless ways to work with our communities and fight the effects of cancer. Each STINGCANCER school is at a different stage of existence and therefore is doing great things, but only doing things that are manageable for their specific group.

To help you brainstorm some fundraising ideas, here is a list of some of the events we have completed:

STINGCANCER Events

- Wear Yellow Day - to show support of cancer patients nationwide
- Children with Cancer Christmas Party
- Charity sponsored run/walks
- Remembrance Day
- Preble Memorial Garden
- Saint Baldrick's events
- Chemo "treat" bags for area oncology clinics
- Locks of Love/Wigs for Kids
- Band-Aid Drive for pediatric oncology
- Gift drive for oncology patients
- Speakers at our meetings
- Yard work/snow shoveling for cancer patients
- Area STINGCANCER Leadership Conference
- And more....

It is exciting for me to share the STINGCANCER idea in this book – a book I believe can truly change your life. Yes, that is what I said: Change your life! That's a powerful statement, but STINGCANCER is a powerful thing.

The challenge to you is this: Keep an open mind and don't be afraid to change. Don't be afraid to add this to your plate. It will be worth it, as you will find immediate fulfillment and success. You will discover STINGCANCER for what it truly is, a journey filled with endless rewards.

Most people have thousands of reasons why they cannot do what they want to do, when all they need is one reason why they can. Your one reason is to change the lives of others – and change your own at the very same time. That is powerful.

Ordinary people like you and me with a strong commitment can make an extraordinary impact on our world. Trust me. I have experienced this first hand.

Together, We Can STINGCANCER!

STINGCANCER
Testimonials

Alex Vernon, senior at Green Bay Preble High School (Class of 2014):

"Monday, February 22, 2010. I arrived at Edison Middle School and walked into the building and gathered by my friends, only to hear the devastating news of the passing of Brittany Cayemberg. Brittany was a sophomore at the time, and her sister was in my eighth-grade class at Edison. The news spread throughout the community and the grief was felt by everyone. I remember hearing about Preble's STINGCANCER group and how big of a difference they had made on the family and Brittany's fight. It amazed me how there was a group like this at Preble and I was interested in making a difference myself.

"Ever since the group was established at Green Bay Preble by Mr. Nick Nesvacil in 2004, STINGCANCER has been Preble's signature organization and an accomplishment we at Preble are proud of. Over 19 schools have joined our mission to STINGCANCER and the numbers are growing. Eventually, STINGCANCER hopes to expand to the collegiate level and broaden its efforts to have an even greater impact. At Preble, STINGCANCER provides a place for students affected by cancer to come together in a setting of hope. We work at community events to raise money for cancer-fighting efforts, as well as annual internal school events that raise awareness for the many needs of cancer patients. Wear Yellow

Day, a day started by Preble STINGCANCER that raises awareness by the color yellow, has become a state-wide day full of hope and awareness.

"To continue on with STINGCANCER's efforts, I plan on establishing a STINGCANCER group at the University of Wisconsin-Stout, my college of choice. I believe the spark that this group has lit inside of me can be lit inside of anyone. I hope to expand the STINGCANCER group throughout colleges around the state, as well as nationally.

"By starting this organization, Mr. Nesvacil provided a forum where togetherness and hope come together and provide a foundation of support for not only people affected by cancer, but to Preble High School as a whole. This club has provided our student body, staff members and alumni something to be extremely proud of. One mission, one goal, one job: working together to STINGCANCER."

"The only place success comes before work is in the dictionary."
- Vince Lombardi

~

Tammy and Brian Charlier, parents of a STINGCANCER member Megan Charlier, who came up with the idea for the STINGCANCER Dinner Gala:

"Mr. Nesvacil, as parents and students involved in STINGCANCER, we are in awe of this fantastic program you have developed at Preble. We believe that its benefits are two-fold: First and foremost, you have brought together a group of students and staff members who share a common bond. Unfortunately, they most likely have been affected by cancer at some point in their lives. The STINGCANCER group allows the Preble community an opportunity to collectively share their experiences with this horrific disease.

"It has helped them form new friendships, but more importantly for many, it has been a form of grief support. Our two children, who had lost their only grandmother to lung cancer, were immediately drawn to this club. It became a source of comfort and solace for them that we, their parents, had never even realized they still needed.

"For this, we thank you Mr. Nesvacil and the STINGCANCER group. Lastly, and equally important, it has provided us all with an opportunity to reach out to others who are experiencing the devastating effects of cancer. The STINGCANCER group brainstormed ideas and activities that would allow them to raise money as well as awareness for the many people suffering from cancer.

"Through their support and caring, they were able to raise money with their Family Fun Day and the STINGCANCER Benefit Dinner. While attending the dinner, it was evident to us what a marvelous group of people the Preble STINGCANCER group is. They were quite proud of their many accomplishments, and those in attendance - parents, spouses, family members, cancer victims and cancer survivors – were overwhelmed with pride for all of them.

"So again, we say with sincerity thank you, Mr. Nesvacil and the Preble STINGCANCER group, for providing all of us with this invaluable experience. Best wishes to all of you as we move forward with STINGCANCER."

~

Wendy DeKeyser, Former Student Counselor at Preble High School who was diagnosed with cancer after writing this. She has since passed away:

"I think the Preble STINGCANCER group has touched more people than we are even aware of. Just the increase in the group's size, alone, each year speaks for itself. Word has spread, and it is all positive. Students, faculty and community want to offer support in some way or another.

"Your STINGCANCER group has offered me hope, and I feel closer to my dad who has died of cancer recently. I am proud to wear the apparel, too! Please let me know if I can ever be of any future help. I think you are doing a great service, Nick. Thank you!"

~

Jenny Olson, a Special Education Teacher at Preble High School:

"In my short time so far here, I believe that the group brings awareness and sensitivity around a subject that people often don't pay attention to unless they are directly affected by it. Here are some things that I feel: It involves many different types of kids. Your group also helps out families in need and shows the importance of compassion. It brings about a sense of community and helps students and adults to see the bigger picture in life. Way to go, STINGCANCER!"

~

Heather Piontek: Deaf and Hard-of-Hearing Teacher at Preble:

"From selling apparel to making signs to raising money, the STINGCANCER group teaches students about how our character counts. Using the group's funds, they are able to make a difference for families in need. Those who suffer from cancer in our community know that they are not alone. Cancer affects all of us. Students who participate in the STINGCANCER group at Preble can see how they can help make the world a better place, simply from the acts of kindness that they do for others affected by cancer. More importantly, it shows them how we are all connected. Great job, STINGCANCER!"

~

Nick Marcelle: Social Studies Teacher and Coach at Preble:

"Everyone can identify with this group. Everyone knows someone who is affected by cancer in some way, shape or form. It is one of the only student groups that has students from all backgrounds. It is a blend of students, who despite different interests, come together for one common cause."

~

Stephanie Smith – Former Special Education Teacher and Co-Advisor of STINGCANCER:

"Nick, it's been a pleasure to be a part of a group such as STINGCANCER. As one of the faculty advisors of STINGCANCER, it has been very rewarding to watch it grow over the past ten years. In the beginning, students were hesitant to get involved and were not quite sure how to contribute to the fight against cancer. Now, our group has grown to over 80 students who are begging for opportunities to help. So many students have emerged as leaders because of being involved in STINGCANCER, and it is fun to sit back and watch these students evolve.

"Preble High School STINGCANCER has also given me hope that there are high school students who are willing to better their community and fight for something they believe in. Too often we hear and see stories about high school students who make poor choices. It is a pleasant change of pace to see students working together for the better of the community.

"On a personal note, when families are faced with fighting cancer they often are left feeling helpless. They want to help, but they don't know how. They want to do something to make it go away, but they can't. Being able to help other families who are dealing with cancer allows me to feel like I am making a difference.

"Nick Nesvacil, the founder of STINGCANCER, is a real inspiration to so many. His hard work and dedication to STINGCANCER are what makes it such a successful group. His vision is now the vision of many. He has definitely made a difference in the lives of so many and has contributed to stinging cancer!"

~

Kari Petitjean: Long-time Secretary at Preble High School:

"In my six years at Preble, I have never seen a group that has brought so many students and staff together for such a common cause like STINGCANCER. I can also say that the amount of calls from the outside community is just unreal. We get all kinds of people wondering what they can do to help support your organization, Nick. I feel that you and your group, STINGCANCER, have made such a huge difference for so many people."

~

Lee Stuyvenberg – Preble Former Special Education Department Chair:

"STINGCANCER's success is outrageous. Who would have ever guessed ten years ago that it would have become the significant community support organization that it has developed into? Keep up the good work, best of luck. Thanks for taking this leadership role, Nick."

~

Pat Aziere – Former Special Education Teacher:

"Hi Nick. I must comment on last night's STINGCANCER meeting. It means so much to one of my students to have the support of this group. As you can tell, he is often the left-behind kid because he's never been able to keep up. His younger brother is bigger and stronger and has lots of friends and lots of freedom. For this young man to be part of a school group is huge.

He is a cancer survivor and he gave a speech about his trial with cancer at a young age.

"After he gave his presentation that was so well received by all the kids, two big buys took him over to their table. To hear them say, "We've got your back, man. And here's my phone number. Call me any time you want to talk," really choked me up. I moved away to give them their privacy, but I could tell how happy this student was because they were talking to him. He has never had the support and attention from his peers that he is getting this year. How do you begin to measure the importance of that?"

~

Jessica Wolf – Para professional:

"Nick, I think you've done something amazing at Preble with STINGCANCER. This is a group that staff and students can work together side-by-side for a good cause. So many high school extra-curricular activities are only self-rewarding. This is a club where people make a difference and students can volunteer sincerely without earning service-learning hours. Today we have so many kids volunteering only because they have to and not because they care. But in STINGCANCER, our students and staff have a purpose together. Thanks so much, Nick, for being the founder of an awesome group. You are an extraordinary guy!"

~

Shelly Cayemberg – Brittany Cayemberg's mother:

"Give freely to the world these gifts of love and compassion. Do not concern yourself with how much you receive in return, just know in your heart it will be returned."

- Steve Maraboli, "Life, the Truth, and Being Free"

"After reading this quote, I thought to myself, this describes Preble's STINGCANCER. When Brittany relapsed the first time, I remembered Deanna Sundstrum coming over to the house. She brought Brittany a subscription to a scrapbooking magazine, some scrapbook supplies and STINGCANCER clothing. This brightened her day and actually got her so involved in scrapbooking and card making that it was her hobby that she could do even when she was sick. Her closet became her crafting studio! As the years went on, STINGCANCER continued to support our family with gift cards and student visits.

"When Brittany was in eighth grade, she had her bone marrow transplant and needed to regain her strength in order to get back to school in the fall. STINGCANCER purchased a pink (her favorite color at the time) mountain bike for her. What a wonderful surprise that was! Even better was being asked to be on the advisory team for Preble's STINGCANCER freshman year. I believe this is what kept Brittany going and determined to beat cancer.

"STINGCANCER had been there for her so many times that now it was her turn to give back and she was going to do it with everything she had in her. I BELIEVE she did it. Who can go from a weeklong chemo treatment, home to shower, change into SC clothes to SC fundraiser until 11 p.m.? Only Brittany, with no sign of quitting!

"The best yet was just before her passing and we had opened our house up to anyone who wanted to say goodbye to Brittany. Instead of her shedding tears, she was asking – no, telling people – what they should donate to the STINGCANCER Dessert Gala, as she knew she would not make it. She even had contacted Aaron Routsala from Kohl's Foundation about speaking without Mr. Nesvacil knowing until he called him! The Dessert Gala was a memorable evening as Brittany's younger sister, Alison, was asked to take her spot on the advisory team for Preble's STINGCANCER for the fall. She graciously accepted, so we have been able to participate in STINGCANCER activities for the last four years.

"I am now happy to say that the elementary school I teach at will be starting a STINGCANCER group in the fall and I can't wait to help them with whatever it is I can do. Nick, you have given so much love and compassion through STINGCANCER. STINGCANCER has taught so many young adults the true meaning of giving that they may have never learned from anyone else. Please know in my heart how appreciative I am for STINGCANCER."

About the Author

Nick Nesvacil survived brain cancer and other major health challenges while in college to become a successful teacher and football coach at Preble High School in Green Bay, Wisconsin. Despite warnings that the chances of fathering any children were slim following his intense cancer treatments, Nick and his wife, Maureen, today are parents to four "little miracles."

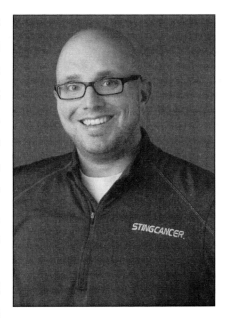

Mike Roemer photo

Nick's cancer journey convinced him of the value that emotional and material support is for patients and their families. He was inspired to create STINGCANCER, a rapidly expanding student-driven support group with chapters in dozens of schools.